W9-CKL-117

The Souvenir

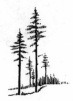

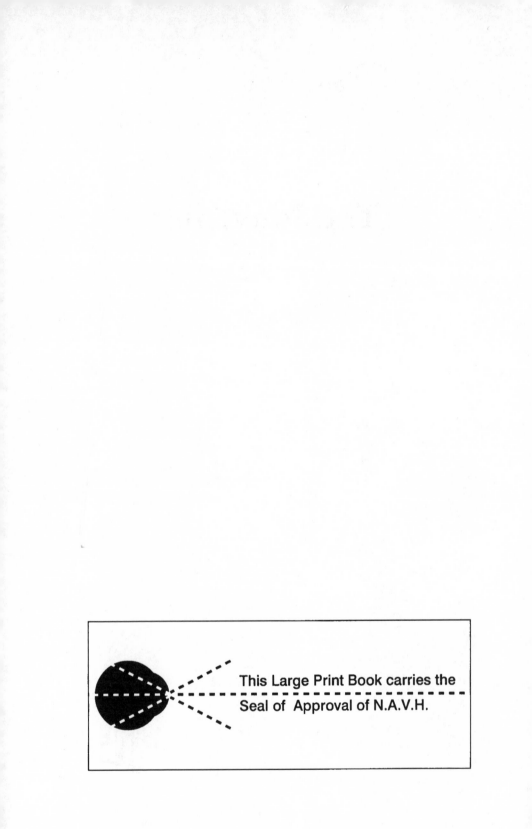

This Large Print Book carries the
Seal of Approval of N.A.V.H.

THE SOUVENIR

A Daughter Discovers Her Father's War

Louise Steinman

Thorndike Press • Waterville, Maine

© 2001 by Louise Steinman.

All rights reserved.

Published in 2002 by arrangement with Algonquin Books of Chapel Hill, a division of Workman Publishing Co., Inc.

G.K. Hall Large Print Core Series.

The text of this Large Print edition is unabridged.
Other aspects of the book may vary from the original edition.

Set in 16 pt. Plantin by Rick Gundberg.

Printed in the United States on permanent paper.

Library of Congress Cataloging-in-Publication Data

Steinman, Louise.
   The souvenir : a daughter discovers her father's war / by Louise Steinman.
      p. (large print) ; cm.
   ISBN 0-7862-3946-8 (lg. print : hc : alk. paper)
   1. Steinman, Norman, 1915–1990. 2. United States. Army —
Biography. 3. Pharmacists — United States — Biography. 4. World
War, 1939–1945 — Biography. 5. United States. Army. Infantry
Division, 25th — Biography. 6. World War, 1939–1945 —
Campaigns — Philippines. 7. World War, 1939–1945 —
Japan. 8. Steinman, Louise. 9. Steinman family. 10. Large type
books. I. Title.
U53.S74 S74 2002
940.54′25—dc21   2001057778

To the memory of my parents,
Anne Weiskopf Steinman (1919–1990)
and Norman Steinman (1915–1990)

The sorrow of war inside a soldier's heart was in a strange way similar to the sorrow of love. It was a kind of nostalgia, like the immense sadness of a world at dusk. It was a sadness, a missing, a pain which could send one soaring back into the past.

Bao Ninh, *The Sorrow of War*

CONTENTS

PART III — The Philippines

PART IV — Suibara

CHRONOLOGY

7 December 1941 Japanese attack U.S. Pacific Fleet anchored in Pearl Harbor, Honolulu, Hawaii.

8 December 1941 Japanese planes bomb Philippine city of Baguio in northern Luzon.

11 March 1942 General Douglas MacArthur retreats from Corregidor, Philippines, after declaring, "I shall return."

August 1943 Newly drafted Private Norman Steinman arrives at Camp Fannin, Tyler, Texas, for infantry training.

January 1944 Private Norman Steinman ships out from San Francisco, crosses the Pacific to join Twenty-fifth "Tropic Lightning" Infantry Division in Auckland, New Zealand. Assigned to Headquarters Company, First Battalion, Twenty-seventh Infantry Regiment "Wolfhounds."

Late February 1944 Twenty-fifth Division lands at Noumea, principal city New Caledonia, for further combat training. "Tropic Lightning" expected to return to fighting lines in June.

June 1944 Tactical plans change. Twenty-fifth remains on New Caledonia for more training. Rehearsals for landing on beaches in Luzon Campaign.

7 December 1944 Twenty-fifth Division convoy, known as Task Unit 77.9, moves out of Noumea, New Caledonia.

21 December 1944 Tetere Beach, Guadalcanal. Twenty-fifth Division stages "dress rehearsal" for landing at Lingayen Gulf.

11 January 1945 Private First Class Norman Steinman lands with Twenty-fifth Division at Lingayen Gulf, northern Luzon, Philippine Islands. Landing unopposed by Japanese troops.

12 January to 10 February 1945 Central Plains phase of Luzon Campaign, including battle for Umingan.

10 February to 21 February 1945 Redeployment and readying for coming assault in Caraballo Mountains of northern Luzon.

3 March 1945 U.S. forces retake Manila from Japanese.

February through June 1945 Battle to secure Balete Pass in Caraballo Mountains, drive from Balete Pass to Santa Fe, and subsequent "mop up" of Japanese hiding out in mountains.

13 May 1945 American forces declare Balete Pass "secure."

16 May 1945 Brigadier General James "Rusty" Dalton of Twenty-fifth Infantry killed in sniper attack while on reconnaissance mission at Balete Pass.

6 August 1945 Atomic bomb dropped on Hiroshima from the *Enola Gay* under orders from President Truman.

9 August 1945 United States drops second atomic bomb on Nagasaki.

12 August 1945 Japanese announce surrender.

15 August 1945 Emperor Hirohito's radio broadcast to his nation asks them to "endure the unendurable."

2 September 1945 Japanese officials formally surrender to Allies aboard U.S. battleship *Missouri* in Tokyo Bay.

2 September 1945 General Yamashita, commander of Japanese troops in Luzon, surrenders to U.S. forces.

24 September 1945 Corporal Norman Steinman and others of Twenty-seventh Infantry Regiment board USS *Natrona* bound for Nagoya, Japan, as part of the U.S. occupation forces.

27 October 1945 After an eighteen-day offshore delay in Wakayama Harbor, Corporal Steinman and other members of the Twenty-seventh Infantry Regiment disembark at Nagoya Harbor.

31 December 1945 Corporal Norman Steinman returns stateside, disembarking in Portland, Oregon, with overnight stay at Vancouver Barracks, Vancouver, Washington.

PROLOGUE

Somewhere at Sea

In January 1944 when my father crossed the Pacific for the first time, he did not know where he was going. He did not know he was headed for New Zealand. He did not know that after a year of training and waiting, first in New Zealand then in New Caledonia, he and his army buddies in the Twenty-fifth Infantry Division would be transported to northern Luzon, the Philippines, where they would sweat out five and a half months of combat.

The monotony, the uncertainty of the destination, the hot sun, the loneliness, the roiling sea all took their toll on him. "I've never felt so blue. It's the thought of leaving you. I hope I can get over it soon, because it's a terrible state of affairs," he wrote to his wife — my mother — from the confines of a transport ship.

As the realization of a long separation sank in — months, possibly years — his mood veered toward panic then settled into depression. Writing letters was his only relief. "Dear Anne," he wrote home, "I'm sorry that you won't hear from me

13

for such a long time until you get this letter, but because of the safety precautions and secrecy involved (for our own good), I wasn't allowed to tell you when I left the States." To describe his location, he wrote simply "Somewhere at Sea" in the upper right-hand corner of each letter.

My father — a graduate of De Witt Clinton High School in the Bronx, with a math degree from New York University — was lacking his usual reference points. No Sunday *New York Times*, no conversations with his parents, no weekly lectures at the 42nd Street branch of the New York Public Library. And the most grievous lack of all — his wife.

It was not like the pragmatic father I knew to daydream, sitting motionless, spinning in his imagination every inch of his wife's body. Her hair. Her smile. The way she wore hats. He composed letters in his mind, wrote them down when the seasickness abated.

　　　　9 January 1944, Somewhere at Sea
Dear Anne,
Since this letter will be censored it is difficult to write. We have already adjusted ourselves to this life at sea. A sailor's life isn't so bad after all.

The first day nearly everyone was seasick. I must admit I was nauseous but I didn't have to feed the fish and it passed very quickly. It was hard to adjust to sleeping in a hammock. But even that isn't so bad when you get used to it. The only thing that none of us can possibly get used to is the congested quarters we live in.

I should have started this letter several days ago but I just couldn't get in the mood to because I was very despondent about leaving and everything that means. Also I knew this letter wouldn't be mailed until we arrived at some port.

I spend almost the entire day on deck, where, when the sun isn't too hot, it is deliciously cool. I keep looking out at the blue ocean and dreaming that you're beside me and, when the moon is out, especially then, I just keep talking to you all the time.

10 January '44, Somewhere at Sea
Dear Anne,
The sun was exceptionally strong today. We were warned not to be exposed in any way to the sun's rays.

I'm sitting on the upper deck gazing out at sea. The wind is whipping at my paper and almost blowing my hat off. Yesterday when I wrote to you, the wind swept one of the pages away.

I'm smoking my corncob pipe and I've just finished dinner. I should be content but I'm still very melancholy. I keep thinking of you so much. I had better pull myself together otherwise I'll be acting like a moron.

The ocean is lovely. It's a deep blue color — almost a navy blue. As the boat moves forward, sometimes small fish fly out of its way. I have seen a large fish — one fellow said it was a shark, but I don't believe that. This just makes me think of the Aquarium in Chicago. I always think of the things we did together. I'm glad we did everything together. You see how my mind works.

As each day goes by, it gives me a very funny feeling to realize how much farther and farther I am sailing away from home. Please believe that I'll be thinking of you constantly. Please have faith in me that I'll come back to you just as soon as the damned war is over.

My heart is heavy but it can't be helped. We just will not be able to see each other for the duration.

You must promise to take care of yourself, because you know how much it will mean to me to know that you are all right.

I love you very much — and I kiss you good night.

The churning motors of the troop ship carried United States Army Private Norman Steinman, serial number 32983436, age twenty-eight, to a latitude farther south than he had ever ventured. Farther from my mother, pregnant with my sister, their first child. Farther from the future he had imagined before the war. Farther from the self he inhabited and could never return to, farther from the person his children would never meet.

And at the same time, the troop ship carried him closer to an enemy he did not know and did not understand — an enemy he was in no hurry to encounter.

PART I

Stateside

CHAPTER ONE

The Pharmacist

"You're not listening," my father used to say when I tried to slip an opinion in edgewise. In any discussion, his was always the last word.

Norman Steinman was a patriarch. Responsible, overburdened, overbearing, tender in his distant way. My father loved to give advice. Even more, he expected to be asked for advice. A Rexall pharmacist, he believed there was a palliative for any kind of illness or physical distress. Emotional distress was not in his purview. His own, he kept private.

Except for some well-worn anecdotes about bossy sergeants and his camaraderie with the characters Captain Yossarian of *Catch-22* and Hawkeye from *M*A*S*H*, he never talked to his children — or anyone else I knew — about his experiences in the Pacific in World War II. He discussed neither his losses nor his sorrows.

In our permissive household, there were few edicts beyond the obvious, like "Stay away from the stove, it's hot." Perhaps that's why the few my parents insisted upon stood out. There were three. The first: Never cry in front of your father. Why? "It reminds him of the war." The second: Never wear black in your father's presence. Why? "It reminds him of his sister, Ruth, who died when she was fourteen." The third: Don't question these rules. Though debate and questions were encouraged in our rambunctious household, these givens were so absolute, my three siblings and I simply accepted them. Whatever happened to him "over there" in the war was off-limits, like a nuclear test zone.

We were admonished never to provoke my father's anger — infrequent but explosive. We were told it was a function of his fatigue. When he was angry or depressed, a familiar and untouchable bad feeling permeated the house. Usually, he just smoldered, but on those occasions when he blew his top, the household froze in its tracks until he retired to his room and slammed the door with reverberating force.

Our doting Russian grandmother used to sigh and say, "The war changed your father. He never had a temper before the war." I never tried to imagine what Norman Steinman was like before the war changed him, or just how this change might have occurred.

After his big heart attack, when he was fifty, my father's doctor advised him to avoid emotional outbursts of any kind. Yet some were as unavoidable as they were inexplicable. One night my mother served him sauerkraut, and he threw the whole plate against the wall. "Something to do with the war," she mumbled as she cleaned up the mess. The mere smell of "Oriental" food made him nauseous. "Reminds him of the Philippines," my mother whispered. The whistling tea kettle was banned from our kitchen. The hissing sound unnerved him. Again, "something to do with the war."

Were it not for a chance discovery, my father's silence about the war might have accompanied him to his grave. While cleaning out my parents' condo in 1991, after my father and then my mother died, I unearthed a metal ammo box from a storage locker in the underground garage. Inside were hundreds of letters my father wrote home to my mother from the Pacific War. In one of those envelopes was a Japanese flag with handwritten characters inked across its fragile face.

These letters, this flag, propelled me on a circuitous, decade-long journey that challenged me to learn more about my father and the men of his generation who fought in the Pacific. To the question, What was Norman Steinman like before he went to war? I would find some answers. But new mysteries would also reveal themselves.

In the decades after he returned home from the Pacific, my father's attention, like that of so many others of his generation, was focused on building a business, providing for his family. He opened his first pharmacy in 1951. Pinned to the bulletin board over my desk is a black-and-white

23

snapshot that shows my parents standing behind the counter on opening day.

They were in their thirties, younger than I am now. My father looks dapper in his white druggist's smock. My mother wears a shirtwaist dress and pearls. They had followed his parents west from New York City after he was demobbed from the army in 1946. They were both eager to raise their children in the bright California light. Wanting a fresh start, my father attended the University of Southern California School of Pharmacy courtesy of the GI bill. My mother ran the house until the youngest of her four was junior high age, and then she embarked on a twenty-year career as a Head Start teacher.

Small and stalwart, my parents both smile into the camera. A banner behind them — OPEN SUNDAY 9 A.M. TO 9 P.M. — testifies to my father's impossibly long hours. In the early years of establishing his business, he worked twelve hours a day, seven days a week. Most nights, he came home and went straight to bed, waking an hour later to eat supper alone. Displays of Ace combs and Gillette razors, Crest toothpaste, laxatives, and a zany pair of giant cardboard spectacles with the phrase "Look to Us!" surround the beaming couple.

In the fifties, Edwards Rexall Pharmacy, my father's store on Sepulveda Boulevard in Culver City, was the hub of our family's well-being and a regular hangout for the neighborhood. (The business came with the name Edwards but we never found out who he was.) The regulars parked themselves in the chrome armchairs by the back counter, airing and comparing their malaise. Those without prescriptions consulted with "Doc" Steinman. He recommended tranquilizers for the nervous rabbi, Kaopectate for the wife of the high school principal, Vi-Daylin to pep up Mr. Alfano from the Villa Italian restaurant next door. A "cousins club" — one large extended family including new arrivals from Kiev and Buenos Aires — received discounts on aspirin, cosmetics, antibiotics.

My siblings and I all worked in the store at one time or another. My after-school job was counting pills from large brown bottles into smaller dark bottles in the back room. Kenny, my younger brother, delivered prescriptions in the red Corvair, dreading the nursing homes where skinny arms reached out to touch him. My older brother, Larry, often worked the counter. "When men wanted to buy condoms, they used signals," he recalls. "Two fingers on the counter, like legs apart." My sister, Ruth, wrapped boxes of Kotex sanitary napkins in plain brown paper before arranging them on the shelves. Reticence and modesty were the era's reigning virtues.

At least once a week we drove over to my grandparents' apartment building, twenty minutes by car. On the way, I always marveled at the giant painted "sky" movie backdrop on the MGM lot. As wide as a football field, this "sky within the sky" could be daylight blue, twilight gray, sometimes inky black. Culver City was the "Heart of Screenland," and illusion was the hometown product. Sniffling movie stars dispatched limos to my father's pharmacy. He loved to tell us how he'd advised Woody Allen to take Chlor-Trimeton. ("He was all stuffed up, a terrible cold. A real gentleman.")

Aside from nitro pills for his heart, my father seldom took as much as an aspirin himself. Nevertheless, he believed in drugs for everyone else. He dispensed Preludin to Ruth for her diets, Benadryl to his wife for hay fever, and Ritalin to me when I needed to pull an all-nighter to study for European history finals. After supper, while I watched *Mickey Mouse Club*, he ordered from the McKesson Company, chanting those magical names into the phone: "One only Phenobarb, two only Doriden, four only Librium, one dozen Penbritin, four ounces paregoric."

The man had an uncanny ability to reduce any situation to its pharmaceutical implications. In 1988, he surveyed my proposed wedding site in Topanga Canyon, north of L.A., noted the blooming chaparral, and soberly proclaimed, "Everyone will need Seldane."

If you felt sick, you were expected to "take something." If you refused to help yourself, he'd cross his arms, sigh, wait out an effective pause, and grumble those dreaded words: "Then suffer." It always worked. If you refused to take something he recommended, you were then be-

26

yond the realm of his protection, the safe haven that only Western medicine and a strong rational father could provide.

By the mid-fifties, my parents owned their own home, a boxy stucco three-bedroom house at 4045 Harter Avenue, a nearly treeless Culver City street lined with similar postwar single-family houses. An eggplant-purple Oldsmobile sedan was parked in the driveway. The centerpiece of the all-concrete backyard was the small built-in swimming pool where Ruth, who'd contracted polio when she was six, could swim to strengthen her limbs.

Every four years or so, my father replaced the family car with a new model, a badge of membership in the postwar consumer adventure. He *always* bought American. The night he arrived home from work in the new Olds, or Ford, or Mercury, was as close as our family ever came to a spontaneous holiday. "Can we go for a drive?" we'd all squeal. And Norman, proud as punch, still in his pharmacy smock, would take his brood for a spin, past the Big Doughnut and the Rollerdrome, the Little League field, the Culver Municipal Plunge.

My father worked long hours so that my siblings and I could attend summer camp, so that my brilliant older brother could take special math and science classes, so that my sister had the best in orthopedists, physical therapy, leg braces. His earnings paid as well for the adjunct helpers to our growing household. Mr. Smith, the pool man, a tall, lanky redhead from Oklahoma, who parked his battered pickup once a week in front of our house, unlatched the gate to the pool yard, and with his long-poled nets expertly scooped dead bugs from the turquoise-hued water. Bessie Greggs, a wry, wisecracking black woman who made the world's best BLTs, came three times a week to help with the housekeeping. A nervous Israeli named Raul tutored my brother in Hebrew. Once a week a handsome Nisei man — nicknamed Porky — mowed the modest lawn and clipped the boxwood hedges. My father respected Japanese Americans, who had served as interrogators with his division in the Pacific.

Porky brought vegetable seeds, and together we'd plant rows of carrots. He showed me how to transplant begonias, aerate lilies. I would kneel beside him and crumble the soil with my hands. He wore a battered khaki porkpie hat that shielded the deep wrinkles in his sunburned brow. My mother told me Porky's family had been in a camp during the war. The camp, with the exotic name Manzanar, was not in Germany, but in California. I was astonished. How could that be?

I'd heard about the concentration camps in Europe. I solemnly observed my parents' choked-up references to nameless relatives "who didn't make it out of Poland or Russia."

One night when I was eight, my mother, who had never forced me to do anything, stormed into the dining room and switched the TV channel from *Zorro*. I protested. Don Diego was on the verge of rescuing a hapless señorita. Mother insisted I sit and watch what was on the screen. Her sternness alarmed me. I didn't budge.

It was a documentary about the liberation of the camps in Europe. Eisenhower was there, wearing a greatcoat, walking slowly past bony men with hollow eyes. White bones and ashes poured out of ovens. Piles and piles of shoes. A mound of human hair. I didn't want to watch, but I couldn't stop looking. Bodies dumped off wheelbarrows into open pits. An arm askew. Faces of the living without expression. A strange sound grew louder than the announcer's somber voice — Mother's stifled sobs.

That night, gaunt bodies pursued me in dreams. The earth yawned open, huge dogs herding my family toward the chasm. The next day at school, I took odd and spontaneous revenge — ripping the pages on Hitler out of the encyclopedia.

It went without saying that nothing made in Germany was ever to be brought into our home. Not even those lifelike Gund stuffed animals I admired at FAO Schwarz. Those hip Volkswagen beetles my friends drove in the sixties elicited my parents' disgust. They also refused to buy Japanese goods — though that made little impression on me. Back then, MADE IN JAPAN was a joke, anyway. You opened the box, the toy fell apart.

As a young child, I was aware of the visceral horror of the Holocaust. By contrast, the Pacific War was distant and vague. There were no books, no photos that impressed upon me the barbarity of the campaign my father fought in northern Luzon against the Japanese. I saw no documentaries about emaciated American POWs in Burma or Bataan, no images of mass suicides of civilians on Okinawa. True, there was the other "H" — Hiroshima — that blasphemy tied to the anxiety hanging over us. But I never made the connection between that tragedy and my father's unmentionable experiences in the war.

I absorbed the general notion that my father had fought a war to make our world on 4045 Harter Avenue in Culver City safe from fascism and military dictatorship. And — at least until the Cuban missile crisis in 1962 — it did feel safe.

I never doubted that my parents loved us, but I was slow to realize how they sacrificed their personal pleasure to ensure the well-being of their children. Our well-being *was* their pleasure. From time to time, my mother gently reminded us how hard Dad was working. Now, when I compare memories with Ruth, it's obvious that he was depressed. "So melancholy," she recalls. "Something was eating him up from the inside."

That I knew so little about Norman Steinman's inner life, or even that he had one, was as much a function of a child's self-involvement as it was a function of the blackout on his emotional history.

I had no idea back then why he longed for normalcy, for quietude, for a small town like Culver City. I had no idea what a feat it was to make a home, a life, and a world of possibilities for your children. I did not yet understand why my father believed if there was a cure for what ailed you, why suffer?

CHAPTER TWO

The Flag

My father lived the last two decades of his life as a cardiac cripple, but he was secretive about the extent to which he suffered from angina. He avoided cold climates, restricted his exercise, never tossed a baseball with his youngest son. He'd furtively slip a vial of nitroglycerin out of his pocket and put a tiny pill under his tongue whenever it got cold, whenever he walked more than a block, after eating a big meal. He reached for that vial by the ocean: he took it out after climbing the steps to my apartment. Since I thought of the nitroglycerin as a last resort, his dependence on it alarmed me, but he'd just wave me off, irritated. He was a prime candidate for bypass surgery or angioplasty, but the truth was the pharmacist was wary of doctors and feared invasive procedures.

I was in New York when my father died in Los Angeles in 1990. Later, I learned that he had not felt well the whole week prior, but he had stubbornly refused to see his cardiologist. Finally, when he couldn't hide the pain from the angina, my mother convinced him to go to the hospital.

"Don't drive so fast," he scolded her. "It's not a matter of life or death."

In the emergency room, he took off his watch and pulled his wallet out of his back pocket. He handed them to my mother. "He knew," she told me. "I could tell by the fear in his eyes." The nurses drew the curtains. The doctors applied the shock paddles, but he was gone.

It was three A.M. in Manhattan when my friend Wendy, a wraith in her long white nightgown, glided into the guestroom and gently shook me from a sound sleep. "Lloyd called. Call him right away." I dialed my husband in Los Angeles.

Had this really happened? My father had suffered his first heart attack twenty-six years ago, when he was just fifty. He had always lived in fear of the next one, but I felt completely unprepared for his loss.

By the time I arrived at my parents' condo in Los Angeles, my siblings were already gathered there. My usually ebullient mother was in shock. The portly upstairs neighbor wheeled in a shopping cart containing two boiled chickens and a pot of broth. My father had always hated this good neighbor's soup.

Ruth and I ordered platters of turkey, pastrami, ham from the deli around the corner. My mother set out pastries and cake, made huge pots of coffee. Relatives — Russians, Argentineans, former Brooklynites residing in the San Fernando Valley — all crowded in.

33

My father, reliably unsentimental, once explained to me his version of the origin of the wake. "In the old country," he said, "people traveled long distances on horseback and in carriages. It was too far to go back the same night. They expected to be fed."

For the rest of the afternoon, whenever any of the cousins or neighbors looked chilly, my mother instructed Larry or Kenny to bring one of my father's jackets from his closet. In the pockets of every one of his jackets was a vial of nitroglycerin. "Enough to blow up the whole building," Larry, the doctor, said grimly. He flushed all the nitro down the toilet.

Larry and Kenny stepped boldly into the patriarchal breach. They decided on a traditional Jewish burial even though our father was not observant. He would be bathed, wrapped in a linen shroud, and buried in a plain pine coffin. Anonymous men, religious Jews, would be paid to sit by his body during the night and sing psalms.

I wanted to see my father one last time. Kenny cautioned me: "He won't be embalmed. He won't look good. His ears are blue." The grief counselor at the Garden of Eden mortuary also considered the request unusual. However, for a fee, the mortuary agreed to prepare him for a last visit.

Lloyd and I drove across town to the Garden of Eden. It was late night in L.A., and even later by New York time. We'd been told the front door to the mortuary would be open. We walked

34

inside; no one was there. The place was eerily quiet. We pushed on the door marked CHAPEL. At the far end of the room, my father lay on a gurney skirted in red velvet pleats and framed by an arch of red velvet curtains.

In life, his personal demeanor had never, even remotely, verged on the theatrical. For this last viewing, however, his naked body was attired in classically draped white sheets. There were two empty chairs beside the body; Lloyd and I both sat down. Kleenex boxes were placed strategically within reach.

It's an animal instinct to want to touch or smell the dead. Elephants tenderly caress with their trunks the carcasses of their kin. Chimps poke at their lifeless companions. Wolves keen. You want to know, with your own senses, that someone is no longer breathing. I kept imagining my father's breath, but he was absolutely still, utterly foreign. I wished I could wrap my arms around him, lay my head on his chest. I willed my hand to stroke his hand, but I could not bring myself to touch him. I wanted to sob, but there was no inner movement, no cracking of frozen feelings.

After an hour, we left the chapel, leaving my father's body alone. In the hallway we encountered a traffic jam of caskets, each with a neatly pressed suit of clothes resting on it. We heard voices and thought we should say we were leaving. One door was slightly ajar. Five Latino mortuary workers were playing poker. As they cut and dealt, they were laughing, drinking tequila, and telling stories. They waved us inside.

I wish we'd taken them up on their hospitality. We both could have used a shot of Sauza Gold just then. My father would have approved; it would have been the right medicine.

From the moment we buried my father, I was gripped with a longing to see him again. To glimpse him on the other side, to see him in a dream. Perhaps I needed reassurance that he'd arrived safely, that he'd assumed new form, even that he was really gone. His departure had been so abrupt, so *final*.

I trailed after short, white-haired men in the supermarket. One Friday night at synagogue, I had to restrain myself from reaching out to caress the nape of the old gentleman sitting in front of me.

The pervasive strength of this desire was surprising. For most of my life, I had taken our differences for granted. Whereas my mother and I were cut from the same psychic cloth, my father and I were made of wholly different material. Or so I always thought.

When I was a kid, on summer visits to New York City, my mother and I used to make a beeline to the Metropolitan Museum. For my mother, who grew up poor, the Met had always been her own private dream mansion. She'd escape the hot tenement on East 11th Street and stroll through the galleries of Greek statues, a woman of leisure alone with classical beauty.

My father's appreciation for art could be summed up by his bringing home a generic Paris-in-the-rain painting from the 1950s equivalent of Wal-Mart, gloating, "It only cost ten bucks." Mother listened to Beethoven string quartets or Verdi arias in the kitchen while she cooked pot roast. My father claimed to be tone deaf.

I never hesitated to confide in my mother. It was standard family policy to spare my father exposure to unpredictable circumstances or raw emotion. "Let's not tell Dad," my mother would say, or, "That would upset your father." Better he be isolated than grapple with difficult feelings.

He was not dictatorial; he allowed his four children their own choices (and their own mistakes). As a teenager, I never had curfews. But when I tiptoed in at three in the morning, my father shuffled through the house in his checkered bathrobe to let me know he was aware of my comings and goings.

I was a child of the psychedelic revolution. I wanted, variously, to be a poet, a dancer, a performance artist, a filmmaker. My coming-of-age was informed by an enthusiastic embrace of hallucinogenic drugs, protests over the war in Vietnam, the draft resistance movement, the emergence of feminism, hitchhiking forays to Big Sur and the Haight.

Growing up in 1960s Los Angeles was rich

with artistic mentors and friendly guides, so I resisted all my father's attempts to offer me instruction of any kind. What could he possibly have to teach me? He wanted to share with me the elegance of quadratic equations; I hated math and tightened up when he supervised my algebra. He wanted me to develop my rational mind. He couldn't fathom why his daughter talked to puppets or spent hours crawling around on the floor of a dance studio, creating performance art pieces few would ever see. No wonder he was always trying to figure out what the hell I was doing. My choices were outside the realm of his experience. He was never indifferent, but was sincerely baffled.

He offered more than once to pay for law school. "If you change your mind," he would begin any conversation about my "career," inevitably infuriating me.

My mother, on the other hand, was always eager to be invited on an escapade. She slept on a box spring with me in a New York City walk-up, shared my unheated room in wintry Wales, a double-seated outhouse on an Oregon commune. I inherited her impulsive nature, a trait both endearing and frustrating to our respective husbands. Her vigor was such a contrast to my father's somber, more plodding tempo. Her bursts of enthusiasm and childlike delight always a contrast to his taciturn, dry wit.

From my perspective, Norman Steinman — who'd worked thirty-five years in his pharmacy

— had excised both risk and introspection from his life. He left the house every morning for his store, filled prescriptions all day, returned at night to the dinner table, his columns of numbers, his bed. The unbuilt world did not call out to him — not the Sierras, not the Mojave, not the California coast. Sleeping in a tent was out of the question. His experiences in the war, whatever those had been, were all the adventure in the Great Outdoors he needed for a lifetime.

"Do you ever think about divorce?" I asked my mother during a spell when it seemed like every word she said irritated him. She looked at me in astonishment. "No, *never*," she said emphatically. Her devotion to my grouchy father was a mystery.

Months passed and my father refused to cooperate. He would not appear in a single dream. His obstinate absence struck me as unfair.

Others arrived and departed without invitation: childhood friends I hadn't thought about in decades; a tap-dancing uncle; Ruth's old boyfriend; neighbors; the janitor from work; the cashier at the neighborhood coffee shop. But my father, for some reason, stayed away.

He paid a dream visit to my mother in the very first week after his death. "He wore a dark suit," she told me, her huge gray-blue eyes wide with astonishment, "and he was holding a hat in his hand. He had a nicely pressed handkerchief in his pocket."

I tried to will him into appearing. I meditated on his image at night before falling asleep, hoping to summon him, but he would not come. I gave up trying, and there were other unforeseen events to deal with. Just weeks after his death, my mother's cancer returned. Three years earlier, she'd had a rare and successful surgery to excise the tumor from her pancreas. Now, nine months after my father's death, my mother was gone. She was seventy-one. At first, I felt a semblance of relief — her physical suffering had been enormous. But she loved being alive. She did not want to die.

"It's a blessing Dad went first," Ruth said grimly. He wouldn't have been able to bear seeing Mother in that kind of pain.

Again the four Steinman siblings and the extended family assembled in the same vault in the same mausoleum in the same cemetery in Hollywood for my mother's funeral. Once again, the relatives convened afterward in the condo. Once again, we ordered platters from the deli. Once again, the upstairs neighbor appeared with the boiled chickens and the pot of broth. Once again, rarely seen cousins told family stories. Why hadn't my father ever told me the names of his ten Russian uncles and aunts? It didn't matter that I was nearly forty years old: I still felt orphaned.

After my mother's death, the bulk of the disagreeable task of dismantling the condominium fell to Lloyd and me. The condo was in a devel-

40

opment with the misleading name Fox Hills. After their four children had grown up and moved out of the house on Harter Avenue, my parents had been ready for a change. For years, my mother had dreamed of moving near the ocean. My father thought the new development, near a shopping center and the airport, was more practical. It was on the first floor, imperative for a heart patient. It was a rear unit, set back from the street, and didn't get much light. He either didn't notice or didn't care. My mother pined for the sun.

With each successive visit, the place felt gloomier. I grew increasingly glum emptying the contents of a kitchen drawer, my mother's bureau, my father's closet. What to do with my mother's rolling pin, boxes of tiny kid gloves? My dad's diploma from pharmacy school, his cuff links, some army medals? Faced with a hodgepodge of family snapshots, I entered a trance, fingering each one. Basically, I was useless. Lloyd labored to pack it all up, exasperated by my inefficiency. I found his workmanlike approach heartless.

The dream of my father did not occur until the following spring, after he'd been dead more than a year. Rain fell, splattering the windows of our upstairs apartment in a sharp staccato.

In the dream I was sick and the weather was lousy. I put on a heavy loden coat my father had given me as a gift. The weight of it made it difficult to breathe or move. Bundled up, I drove my car through the dark city in the pouring rain, trying to find a pharmacy that stocked the cure for what ailed me. I tried a Sav-on, a Thrifty Drug. At each one, the on-duty pharmacist shook his head. Moving on, I saw a pharmacy I'd never noticed before. A storefront, like a relic from the fifties. I ran inside. There behind the counter, wearing his priestly white smock, stood my father.

He was a small man, but in the dream he was huge. He was a gentle man but in the dream he raged. "You haven't visited in months," he hissed. "You've been *ignoring* me." Anger darkened his face. I tried to protest. I'd sat with his corpse in the Garden of Eden mortuary. I'd been to his funeral. I'd seen his pine coffin shoved into the wall. I was *sure* he was dead. None of these excuses placated him. He was livid. He exploded once again: "You've been *ignoring* me. You haven't been *listening.*" His rage broke against me like a wave.

Before dawn, I woke up terrified, listening to the sound of pounding rain.

Two weeks after the dream, Lloyd and I were finally close to finishing the seemingly interminable task of clearing out the condo. We taped some boxes shut and prepared to leave. Then I remembered the storage locker in the underground garage. We took the elevator down. An unmarked key on the key ring opened the

42

padlock to the locker.

In the dim light, I identified a collection of odds and ends. A motley box of my old theater props, a spare soup pot, Grandma's everyday dishes, two frayed beach chairs, a bicycle missing a front tire. At the bottom was a rusted metal ammo box. I tried to pick it up, but it was too heavy. I tried to open it, but the hasp was stiff. We hauled the box toward the light and together pried it open. I had a vague memory of having seen this artifact once before. Inside the rusted box were stacks of yellowing airmail envelopes. These were all addressed to my mother in my father's handwriting. Hundreds of them. The faded dates on the envelopes spanned 1941 to 1945.

Under one bundle of letters was a manila envelope postmarked March 3, 1945, and stamped on the back with some kind of an official seal:

Pursuant to provisions of War Dept. Memo W/370-3-43, 22 July 1943, and of Headquarters, USAFFE Circular No. 21, 5 March 1944, the bearer Norman Steinman PFC 32983436 of this certificate is entitled to retain in his possession or to mail the following: 1 Japanese flag.

I opened it and found a slippery piece of white silk, folded in eighths. I held it up to the light. Pin pricks of daylight showed through the fragile fabric — tiny holes where the fine strands had given way. The orange-red disc in the center was faded. Brushed over the surface were Japanese characters, and speckled among them, faint drops of red-brown. Could they be blood? Spooked, I quickly refolded it and put it back in the envelope, back in the box.

Months later, after we finally sold the condo, I brought the ammo box and its contents home to my apartment. The letters, by their sheer quantity, were intimidating. They lay in their inelegant sarcophagus like a reproach. The abundance of them was alarming. When I occasionally plucked one out to read, it always had the same effect, detonating a landmine of longing for my father. The flag remained in its manila envelope buried under the piles of correspondence, too disturbing to contemplate.

However, as time wore on, a shift occurred. The contents of the metal box, which had initially frightened me, now began to draw me in. At odd moments, I'd pull the box out from the closet and read a few letters. I noted a cast of characters — "Dr. Orange," Hal Rubin, Morrie Franklin, someone named Sam Wengrow. Who were they? I began to realize that the metal box contained a story, many stories. Tales of fear, bravery, and kindness, the mundane and the heroic intertwined.

I'd take out the flag and examine it, running my hands gently over its shimmery surface, folding it up and placing it back in its envelope. For months it didn't occur to me that the Japanese characters actually meant anything. They were just mute forms, swirling across the surface of the silk.

One day, on a seemingly mindless impulse, I searched through my Rolodex at work. My job then was at an underfunded city arts center, coordinating theater and dance programs. I found the telephone number of a Japanese performance artist named Rika Ohara.

I didn't explain to Rika why I needed to see her, but she agreed to come to my office anyway. She was a striking young woman. Her head was shaved, and her delicate features were not disguised by the loose-fitting slacks and oversized flannel shirt she wore. Her thumb and forefinger were stained tobacco-yellow. She was one of the few who still rolled her own smokes.

We sat outside on a bench, shaded from the sweltering sun. I opened the envelope and gently pulled out the flag. "I found this with my father's things after he died," I said. "He fought in the Philippines. He must have found this on a battlefield." She looked at the flag but didn't say a word. "I'd like to know what these characters mean," I said. She listened but she didn't answer right away.

I sat holding the flag on my lap as Rika plucked tobacco from a tin and placed it precisely on the crease of a cigarette paper. She daintily moistened the gummed edge, then formed it quickly into a smoke. She placed it in

45

her mouth and lit up. Then she glanced up from her task and took the flag from me in her small fine hands.

She looked at it silently for what seemed like a long time. Whatever she was thinking, she didn't let on. Perhaps I should defend my interest in this ghoulish artifact, I thought. I didn't know how my father had come to have the flag. I refused to assume the obvious: that he'd taken it off a dead soldier. Yet I felt a rush of shame.

Finally, her fingertips still caressing the flag as if she were reading Braille, Rika turned to me and said, "This is a good-luck banner, given to a Japanese soldier when he goes into battle. Perhaps when he leaves for duty overseas. It says here: 'To Yoshio Shimizu given to him in the Greater East Asia War — to be fought to the end. If you believe in it, you win.' That's what it says. The other characters on the flag are names." She gingerly handed the flag back to me. Her cigarette had gone out. She calmly lit up.

I wanted to ask my father about the flag, about Yoshio Shimizu. Norman Steinman didn't know his enemy had a name. And, I was pretty sure, he wouldn't have wanted to know.

CHAPTER THREE

Into the Deep

Among the mementos I found with my father's letters was a wallet-size membership card in something called the Domain of Neptunus Rex.

The card reads:

DOMAIN OF NEPTUNUS REX

TO ALL SAILORS, whoever ye may be, and to all Mermaids, Sea Serpents, Whales, Sharks and other Living Things of the Sea, GREETINGS;
KNOW YE that on this day there appeared one

Norman Steinman

who, having invaded our Royal Domain by crossing the Equator on the U.S.A.T. SF #1650 has been, and is hereby, gathered to our fold and initiated into the Solemn Mysteries of the Ancient Order of the Deep.

GIVEN, UNDER OUR HAND AND ROYAL SEAL, this
12th day of January, 1944.
Neptune I, Rex Ruler of the Raging Main and
Davy Jones, His Majesty's Scribe

After a week at sea en route to New Zealand, my father noted, "Today we crossed the Equator and we had a Father Neptune party on the deck and it was really good." I imagined a scene of levity: a GI with a long white beard dressed in fishnet stockings parading around the deck of the transport ship with a trident, while thirty or forty seasick doggies — that's what they called themselves (doggie for dog-faced, expressionless) — hooted and hollered despite their discomfort.

After months of training in Tyler, Texas, the GIs were finally on their way to "the real thing," to the war itself. The satiric Neptune ritual, that shipboard frivolity, was a sanctioned way to release the tension of a long journey. But the vaudeville that celebrated the first crossing into a lower latitude masked a more somber initiation. The "membership card" was supposed to mark the end of life as these soldiers knew it; certainly life as my father had known it. Combat would actually effect the most profound transformation in these men's lives. Combat would initiate them into a fraternity of men both ancient and silent; the fraternity of men who have faced death — who have killed or been killed in war.

About male initiation rituals, the scholar Mircea Eliade writes, "When the boy comes back from the forest . . . he will be another; he will no longer be the child he was. He will have undergone a series of initiatory ordeals which compel him to confront fear, suffering and torture, but which compel him above all to assume a new mode of being." In my father's letters, as well as evidence of change, I would find evidence of who he was before the war changed him.

The soldiers threw scraps of food from their King Neptune celebration over the railing to the dolphins and gulls. The other creatures of the deep — the whales, the sharks, the sponges, the rays, the blowfish — scarcely noticed the big boat carrying soldiers to war, casting a temporary shadow on their realm.

In the fall of 1992, a little more than a year after my parents' deaths, I quit the day job I'd had for five years and headed north for a month to a writers' colony at Fort Worden State Park outside the town of Port Townsend, Washington, on the Olympic Peninsula. With me were my husband, my dog, and my father's letters.

I wanted to try to understand the connection between my father's silence about the war and our family's home life. I wanted to understand the ordeals that compelled Norman Steinman to assume a new mode of being.

I figured if I could just lock myself in a cabin with all those letters, I might unravel the narrative of those war years and comprehend some truth about the man, his experience, his pain. I wanted to know *how* the war changed him.

We arrived at Fort Worden late at night and followed the map to our assigned domicile. I'd imagined our living quarters would be one of the fine Victorian officer's houses on the main quad, like the ones in *An Officer and a Gentleman*, which had been filmed here. But cottage #255, originally intended for an enlisted man and his family, was a simple wooden bungalow. Three bare little rooms, a woodstove, some dilapidated furniture.

The next morning Lloyd and I set up my computer in the little office that faced south into the woods, and brought in extra tables to make a modest studio for him in the dining room. Lloyd, a sculptor, would use this time to paint.

I pinned on the wall a large 1945 map of the Philippines I'd found among my father's letters. The principal battles I marked in red: Balete Pass, Luzon, Leyte Gulf, Corregidor. The names of battles were actual physical places. My father had written about some young soldier from Texas named Melvin Smith who was killed in some place called Umingan. Where was Umingan? I located a speck on the map.

I pulled the crumbling rubber band off a clump of letters, opening the now-fragile, yellowing envelopes and V-mails. The creases in the thin paper were well worn.

My mother, until now the only reader of this correspondence, had bundled the letters by month; she'd numbered each letter in sequence — from one to four hundred and seventy-four. I arranged the months within the proper year, and separated the years into different boxes. I established a daily practice of logging the letters, then reading and transcribing them. By typing his words — passing them through my sight into my hands and onto my computer — I began to absorb them.

I noticed how his handwriting varied depending on the time of day (at mealtimes, in between skirmishes), his location (on a bunk, in a hammock, in a foxhole), the quality of illumination (flashlight, candlelight, electric bulb), his writing instrument (fountain pen or pencil), his level of exhaustion and discomfort. What would take longer to grasp was how his own experience fit within the chronology of the Pacific War campaign.

The letters could be divided into four main periods: stateside training (1943, at Camp Fannin in Tyler, Texas); more training overseas (1944, in New Zealand and New Caledonia); combat and its aftermath (most of 1945, in northern Luzon in the Philippines); and the United States Army occupation of Japan (October to December, 1945, on a navy ship and in garrison near Nagoya).

I'd set a goal for a given day, say, transcribe all the letters from December 1944, or half of the letters from January 1945. But once I'd begun, it was difficult to stop. My order would break down and I'd pull letters to read at random out of the boxes. What was February 12, 1944, like? What was happening the second half of June 1945? I'd start in the morning and then look up amazed to see the dusky northwest sky streaked with purple and red.

Knowing that his wife would read what he wrote both consoled my father and gave him the ability to observe what was happening around him more objectively. He also knew to temper his descriptions with reassurance. Her letters to him were a lifeline; in those gaps of time when he was unable to receive them, he suffered. They were constant reminders of a life worth living, a family to come home to, the ongoing daily saga of her life in Brooklyn — these were precious talismans. The constancy of their correspondence was unusual.

22 August 1944, South Pacific
I'm so glad you find my letters to you so satisfying. I have always written how much I enjoy your writing ability. I never realized that I have developed a style of writing of my own. I just write as though I were conversing with you. And these days when I am so on edge, thinking of what you are going through, it is an outlet for me — to keep

writing to you. The lengthier the letter the better I feel. It helps take a little of the tension off me. In between pages I usually pace the floor, then come back and read your old letters and write some more. That process goes on all evening, until I am rescued by Wilbur who gets hungry and decides I have written enough and we ought to eat something.

Even in the stressful period of preparing and waiting to go into combat, he continued to write home.

24 November 1944, South Pacific

I can now see the point of view of the older fellows (older in terms of service). They write very seldom because, when the going gets tough and they don't write at all, their folks at home aren't accustomed to receiving a steady flow of mail, so they don't mind it as much.

But I will continue writing whenever I get the opportunity because that is the way you would want it.

I'm thankful that I have you and Ruth as an inspiration and no matter how tough the going — I'll get back to you both someday. Perhaps sooner than we dare hope we shall be back in each other's arms and look back on this period of separation as a horrible nightmare.

There were periods of weeks, especially later during combat in Luzon, when the mail could not be taken out or brought in to the troops over the rugged mountain trails surrounded by the enemy. During those times, my mother had no way of knowing whether her husband had been wounded or was still alive. Her nerves were on edge, her imagination primed for disaster.

29 April 1945, Philippine Islands

Dearest,

I write tonight with a heavy heart. One of my close friends just went the way of Dr. Orange. He sure was a swell lad — tops in everything. He was one of our old timers. It was he that was expecting the visit from his wife who is an army nurse — and he was the one that I spent many hours tutoring in trigonometry. He had such a burning desire to complete his formal education. I'm so deeply shocked that he is gone. The Grim Reaper of War sure takes his toll and always he picks on the cream of our youth. God how much longer can it go on?

Though subject to army censors, his letters answered a question I had never dared to ask while he was still alive: "What was the war like, Dad?" I began to discover the texture of his experiences — his appetites, longings, fears.

Food was frequently on his mind. He dreamed of Dagwood sandwiches: corned beef, pastrami, rolled beef and salami with relish, cucumbers and pickles. He fantasized about "Italian food at Leone's and Little Venice. Swedish food. Smorgasbord at the Stockholm. French food at Pierre's. Chicken dinner at Mom's and some good American cooking at home from the Settlement Cook Book — a way to a man's heart." My mother sent packages from Brooklyn containing sardines, shrimp, anchovies, olives, and pickled herring, which he shared with his buddies. He noted that her honey cake arrived spoiled. His fatigues were always dirty. His quarters were "miserably hot, comparable to a Turkish bath." Living with so many other men was "similar to a cross-section of Coney Island and the bedlam of Times Square during the rush hours." He longed for the comforts of home.

27 October 1944, South Pacific
Hello Dearest: I've been doing a heap of just plain thinking these days, but really it hasn't been brooding. Mostly I think of little things such as sitting down at a table with real chinaware — and an easy chair with a hassock to put my feet on — and a pipe, pajamas, robe, and slippers — and a rug, a lamp and a beautiful symphony all blended together with you in every thought.

And being able to go to the refrigerator for an ice cold beer — and some fruit — and even chocolate milk — or honestly, just a quart of plain old milk.

Yesterday we were dreaming of a bathroom. How it would feel to step out of a steaming hot shower onto a bathmat — have real running water out of faucets and a real tiled commode and a large mirror to shave — and, I don't have to go on — but it makes me feel better to write it down.

We spend time staring at ads in the magazines that arrive regular mail. I love most the ones that show a tumbler of whiskey and soda with ice cubes in it — and a man wearing a white shirt — and pictures of sport clothes like a plaid shirt. Gosh.

Will you make some ham and eggs when we get back? Real eggs — sunny side up — and not scrambled? Can I mess the Sunday *Times* all over the living room floor before you read it? Can I leave my sneakers all over the house and knock pipe tobacco on the rug?

The booming of the big guns woke him up from sound sleep. Some men did not take off their shoes for a whole month. They slept in all their clothes. They kept puppies and monkeys for pets. "You'll find a monkey in almost every jeep or truck. The boys all like to play with them." When the men bathed they often found themselves encircled by eyes; the native women liked to watch their lean bodies and muscular arms. A skinny white horse wandered through their camp one night, and it was a wonder it was still alive because "they throw grenades at shadows after all."

With a letter written from New Caledonia, he enclosed two pictures of a young doe:

21 October 1944

The boys had caught it and were taking it for a mascot. Then some dumb bastard shot it and wounded it and left it to die.

Our boys found it the next day down the creek, and the medics brought it in on a litter and tried to save its life. They fed it condensed milk with an eyedropper but the doe finally died. The doctor diagnosed it as suffering from shock and loss of blood.

I thought you would like to see the pictures. I did the printing of them. How do you like the workmanship? Not bad for an amateur.

I guess I'm not descriptive enough to relate how the medics worked over the animal and how our whole company was interested in its welfare, always asking for last minute communiqués etc. I hope the two pictures get through.

Between Brooklyn and the Pacific Islands, my parents' letters frequently crossed in the mail. Correspondence lagged, arriving fifteen days late in bunches of three or five. Once the mail was so backed up, my father received thirteen letters from Brooklyn in one day.

On my mother's twentieth-sixth birthday, her father died of stomach cancer in New York's Bellevue Hospital. That same night, she wrote a long letter to her husband, one of the few letters of hers to survive the war.

3 May 1945

Dearest Friend,

I am writing this letter so that I can bare my innermost thoughts, and relieve my pain and sorrow. I may never send this letter to you. Your sorrows are sufficient for you to bear right now, and I can't burden you any more. But I need you desperately — and, well — at least writing helps some.

You see, Norman, today I said goodbye to my father.

I'll never lose sight of the fact that you, too, have seen men die — men who are young, who had every right to live. Perhaps you, yourself, have had many a narrow escape. I know that my father was not a young man. I also know that no man is immortal. Only — Papa did not deserve to go as he did. I'll skip the details, though you are most likely calloused to gruesome sights. The only fortunate phase in the whole tragedy was that Papa was spared being aware. He never knew what was happening. But we did. . . .

Oh! He was a stubborn man! He even died a stubborn death. He was a simple man —

he asked and received very little in life. How he loved children. How he adored his grandchildren. Oh Norman! How he loved your Ruthie! And Papa loved you, Norman. Until the very last, he talked about how he prayed for your homecoming. He did *so* want to see you again.

I'll always remember the relationship between my father and mother. Theirs was a love of years — a love of toil and constant struggle. I'll always cherish the fact that when my father left for the hospital, Mama left out one item when she made a clean sweep of Papa's belongings. She left his trousers hanging in the bathroom just as he had always done. I appreciate that fact for I recall that when I packed your belongings into the trunk, I felt badly. And what I left for last, and hated most, was taking the tie rack down and putting away your ties.

It was twenty-six years ago that I was born unto my parents. I made that day an occasion for my parents. And that date will be forever linked up now.

For on May 3rd, 1945, a date recording my birth — also records the date of my father's death.

And so life goes — Anne

That sad letter crossed with my father's V-mail, written that same day during combat in Luzon, apologizing for forgetting her birthday.

Three weeks later, he still did not know his father-in-law had died.

21 May 1945

Today's letter from my mother tells me your dad is feeling better. Please don't keep anything from me. Let me know how your dad is getting along from time to time. It's better that you tell me all your sufferings rather than keep them all to yourself. Break down to me once in a while; you'll feel better that way.

Not until June 1945, a month later, did he finally write his tender letter of condolence, ending with, "We all have to take the passing of our parents at some time in our lives. It is the most bitter pill to swallow in one's life. And so much harder for you because you didn't have me with you to help share your burden. I hope this letter helps a little."

My father's letters ranged widely in tone. In moments of boredom, lying in a hammock on a troop ship, he offered practical advice: what to say to tactless friends whose husbands weren't away at war, but home making money. Or, words of comfort, reassurance that they would start over once the war ended: "Everything will be different when we move from New York to Los Angeles, the ideal place to raise our family." During his first days of combat in Luzon, in January 1945, he described the appalling conditions that prevailed in a war zone: "My mother told me there would be nights like this! It rained so hard it broke down the stakes supporting our ponchos that were over our holes — our hole began to fill up and we were sleeping in mud. After a while the heat of our bodies made the mud tepid and it was a little more comfortable. The medics cooked some chicken in a helmet — and I had some of it for chow."

After that, something mundane follows: "When you enclose stamps how about putting them in between wax paper — because they are always stuck to the envelope." In February 1945, already combat-hardened, he requested, "Please don't use the salutation 'Hello Angel' in your letters."

The military censor always read over his shoulder. "I have an idea this letter is going to be a very long one. At this stage, the censor must be getting tired," he wrote solicitously at one point.

The censor knew specific things about Private Steinman; he knew, for instance, that he had no respect for the chaplain. ("The Holy Mackerel" he called him, complaining that "the Chaplain is always telling me *his* problems.") The censor knew intimate details: During rifle drill, Private Steinman had been daydreaming about his wife's earlobes. The censor knew that Private Steinman's dreams almost landed him in trouble with his tent mate:

I sleep in a pup tent with a very old regular Army man — my platoon sergeant. He is a swell guy who has been in the Army over ten years. He's in his late thirties. While sleeping this afternoon, I was dreaming of you — and two people in a pup tent are very close to each other — and I had a great desire in my dream to kiss you. It's a lucky thing I woke up just then because I'm sure the sergeant would have doubted me and wondered whether my intentions were honorable.

They both learned to read between the lines. There were code words to elude the censor's eyes. Either my parents had agreed upon them in advance, which is unlikely since they didn't know what combat would be like, or they counted on each other to decipher the meaning in context.

I puzzled over the enigmatic phrase "Hal Rubin's gift" that surfaced so many times, as in "I'm nowhere near where I can get that gift for Hal Rubin." It took me weeks to decode its meaning.

Hal Rubin must have been a friend or acquaintance back home in New York, the kind of pushy guy on the dance floor who'd cut in when you were happily partnering with your wife. Hal Rubin had apparently requested a war souvenir, the kind that could only be procured where there were dead Japanese soldiers around. The name served as a code word for the front lines during combat, and sometimes even for the enemy himself. My father's use of the enigmatic phrase shows how he both dreaded combat, and, conversely, yearned to get it over with.

16 November 1944

Hal Rubin still has several weeks before I can get him the gift that he asked for.

17 November 1944

I'm wondering a lot these days if I ought to get that little gift for Hal Rubin. After all, he never got any for us. If the opportunity presents itself I may — but I've decided not to go out of my way for it.

3 December 1944

I know I've been very incoherent in my letters of recent days but if you are confused please remember that I too am even more confused. And what annoys me most paradoxically is that I have to postpone and wait a little longer to get that damned gift for Hal Rubin. I am very impetuous and don't like waiting, it always puts me on edge. I like to get things done and over with. But I suppose it is for the best.

Somehow I think that you're not a bit angry about the delay and even wonder why I'm making so much of a fuss about the goddamned gift. But it is an outlet for me. I've been in a rut ever since I've joined this army

— and I hate it very much. I want to do something and help get this damned war over with so that I can get back to you and everything dear.

                    12 December 1944
That gift for my pal Hal Rubin may come up pretty soon — and I'm kinda glad that it is. Although I never was really anxious or enthused about the whole thing. I like to get it over with so that I can give it to them, and then relax. I think we've been waiting long enough and I'm tired of waiting. So if you see Hal, don't tell him or anyone about it, because I do want it to be a surprise.

The correspondence I was reading was, however, just a one-sided dialogue. My father had no choice but to destroy most of his wife's letters to him as he moved from place to place. He kept them as long as he could, and read them over and over again.

                    20 March 1945
This business of destroying your letters that I have been saving and of which I was so proud has gotten me down. I can't do more than three at a time before quitting. A wave of nostalgia and lonesomeness seeps over me. It's a very depressing process.

Reading my father's letters brought back

memories. I remembered our walks to buy milk at Taylor's Liquors, around the corner from our house in Culver City. We often passed Mr. Roberts, who wore dirty overalls and muttered to himself. A nervous tic rhythmically distorted his unshaven face. His unkempt son, Michael (who later died in Vietnam), was my older brother's age. His daughter, Freda, was in my fourth-grade class. Nobody would go near Freda. The boys made faces if they had to hold hands with her. No one ever asked her to be on their kickball team or to be their partner for square dancing because Freda, with her dirty hair and rumpled dresses, always smelled like she had messed herself.

Now I remembered how, when we had safely passed, my father admonished me gently. "You should always be nice to Mr. Roberts," he said. "Mr. Roberts is shell-shocked."

That was the first time I'd ever heard the expression "shell-shocked." It made me think of those little chicks I loved to watch in the incubator at the science museum. They pounded their beaks against their shells trying to hatch, then emerged stunned, dripping wet and exhausted. Even as a child I knew that "shell-shocked" had something to do with why Mr. Roberts talked to himself and why his poor daughter smelled so bad. The war had wrecked them both.

I recognized the man in my father's letters by his humor, his steadiness, his logical explanations. But now I encountered a side of the man that he had never revealed to his four children, a side that was passionate, unguarded, emotional, poetic: "Remember how I used to enjoy the beauties of nature, especially the Heavens at night?" he wrote from Luzon to his young wife, "how we used to like a bright moon and a starry sky? Well it's so hard for me to enjoy anything now." I began to understand why he would never camp or hike when I was growing up.

The man who wrote these tender letters was different from the man I had known. My exhilaration at glimpsing my father's former self was tempered with sadness when I understood how the war had sealed off his emotions.

No shots were ever fired from the high cliffs of Fort Worden, where Lloyd and I were staying. During World War II, the soldiers here were battle-ready but never saw combat. They waited. Each day, each night they scanned the sea for the enemy, but the enemy never arrived. The army melted down the big guns for anchors in 1943, and abandoned the fort altogether ten years later.

Now Mother Nature was reclaiming the place. Glimpsed at a distance through the dense foliage, the massive abandoned gun batteries could have been mistaken for Mayan ruins. Iron doors guarded vacant rooms etched with graffiti. Scotch broom and horsetail ferns sprouted between the metal tracks that had once moved cannons.

Behind our cabin were miles of trails criss-crossing the woods of Douglas fir, cedar, and madrone that lead to concrete battle fortifications dug deep into the earth. Every morning we went out, we took different back roads and trails around the fort, our terrier gamely rooting through the underbrush. After our walk, I'd read some more letters.

Norman Steinman was a city boy from the Bronx; the jungle was completely alien to him. So too was darkness.

> 24 April 1945, Philippine Islands
> . . . And in the middle of the night in Stygian darkness where you couldn't see your hand in front of your eyes, I had to creep out of my hole in a downpour and sit behind a machine gun whose field of fire was a trail — and all I could do was sit and listen — and my body was shaking with cold due to the change of temperature of sleeping then sitting up. And the trees made sounds, and the birds jabbered, and the monkeys most of all sounded almost human.

Stygian, from the dark river Styx in Greek mythology, across which all dead souls were ferried to the underworld. My father was writing from the embrace of death, and he would need help to feel the forces of life again.

I waited patiently on our daily walks as Lloyd and our dog enthusiastically explored connecting tunnels and empty concrete vaults. I had no intention of ever going into an abandoned bunker myself. I don't like the dark.

One morning we hiked out to Battery Kinzie at the end of the beach near the old lighthouse. The concrete was stained dark from the rain. Brushstrokes of an antigraffiti campaign, in quasi-camouflage pattern, had taken on a shiny patina over the years. The sun came out. We ran in crazy circles over the broad cement roof of the bunker, staring out over the dunes to the sea, where a tugboat was hauling two huge barges through the choppy Straits of Juan de Fuca. The wind was wicked. My parka was zipped up to my ears.

I noticed a set of stairs disappearing down in the dark. I whistled for Lloyd to come see. I wanted to point out to him how dark it looked down there. He charged down the stairs, dog at his heels, shouting back at me, "C'mon!"

"But I'm afraid of rats," I whimpered. "Nothing here for the rats to eat!" he shouted back, his voice growing fainter the deeper he went. I waited for them to come out. And waited. I felt stupid. I was afraid of going down into a dark tunnel in peacetime while my father had slept in cold mud night after night during combat.

I slowly made my way down into this artificial underworld, cautiously moving into what I sensed to be the center of the crypt. I stopped and panicked. I wanted out. Then it occurred to me to look back at my point of entry. The light from outside was dazzling, framing the stairs in a brilliant white rectangle. When I closed my eyes, the glowing shape was visible through my lids.

I glanced back into the dark with open eyes, and was completely blinded. "Where are you?" I yelled and was startled at the sound of Lloyd's voice just a few feet away. I thought of those monkeys jabbering like crazy humans in the jungle night. I turned and saw the faint glimmer of daylight at the far end and started to walk toward it as fast as I could.

It was then I realized that I could never, really, grasp the fear my father and his fellow soldiers had felt in the jungle. In Luzon, when they sealed the caves dug by the Japanese, the GIs took turns entering the dark caverns all alone. It was incredibly dangerous. They checked for stragglers, then lobbed a grenade and beat a hasty retreat. For months at a time my father had slept with his hand on his rifle, in a hollow in the dirt, struggling against the fear that he would not return home.

We turned back to the cottage and each headed into our respective workspaces. I was relieved to be sitting in the warmth and light of my little office. I could hear Lloyd cursing through the wall as he worked on a painting. I read some letters and began transcribing.

CHAPTER FOUR

A Melancholy Slav

My father was five and a half years old in 1921 when he emigrated to the United States from the town of Zhitomir in Ukraine. He traveled with his seven-year-old sister, Ruth, and his mother, Rebecca. His father, Herschel (American name: Harry), had left Russia a year earlier to lay the groundwork for the family's new life in America. He waited anxiously for the first sight of his wife and children as they arrived on the boat at Ellis Island.

As my grandmother walked down the ramp, with her daughter at her side and her small son's hand held tightly in hers, the immigration officer gestured them aside, pointing to Aunt Ruth's shiny black braids. "I thought he wanted to admire her beautiful hair," my grandmother told me seventy years later, "but instead he told me to untie the bow so he could look for bugs."

I found my grandmother's transit visa from Russia in one of the many dusty boxes in my parents' condo. The yellowing paper was inscribed with sepia ink and stamped by the Polish

Komisar: "Legation De Belgique En Pologne," it reads. Born in "Imperium Rosyjskiego," the Russian empire. The photo on the visa shows my thirty-year-old grandmother, Rebecca, in a high-necked silk dress surrounded by her two children; my father with close-cropped hair and a ruffled sailor collar; my aunt Ruth with her long braids in a modest pinafore and white blouse. The children gaze solemnly into the camera.

I used to pester my father with questions about his childhood in Russia, but he claimed to have no memories at all. If he did, he said, he could not distinguish them from dreams, and he never remembered his dreams. My grandmother, on the other hand, did not hesitate in recollecting the life she had left behind. It was as real to her as the carton of milk on the table. "Do you know, Louisey," she would say, "how we came from Zhitomir?"

"That happened so *long* ago!" my father would admonish the tiny straight-backed old woman. Or he'd say, "Mother — you've already *told* us about that." That was invariably true, but I never got tired hearing her tell the story again. With each telling she added new details, a slight twist of emphasis. She waited until her son left the room, and then resumed her tales.

Except when he was in the army during the war, my father was never separated from his mother. After she was widowed and moved into the Golden Crest Retirement Hotel, he drove across town after work almost every night to visit her. For the last decade of her life, she moved in with my parents. "Your father breathes in; your grandmother breathes out," my mother used to say with a hint of exasperation. When she and my father purchased a crypt at the mausoleum, my mother chose a location two floors above her in-laws. "One lifetime is enough," she quipped.

My father wanted to marry Annie Weiskopf, my mother, from the moment he saw her. She was a precocious, feisty fifteen-year-old. He was nineteen, a student at New York University. They met at a Socialist Party dance. She was struck with the serious, handsome young man with wavy blue-black hair and pale blue eyes, but she was far too young to make a commitment. He courted her for five years, made her agree to date no one else. They married two months before her twentieth birthday, and celebrated with a weekend in the Catskills.

His family was far more prosperous than hers. Grandpa Harry, my father's father, owned a haberdashery in the Bronx. My mother's parents were poor Polish immigrants. Louis Weiskopf, my mother's father, sold newspapers from a stand on lower Broadway. He ran numbers and the gangsters paid him off. Sarah Weiskopf, my maternal grandmother, worked in a bakery and brought home stale cream puffs to add to the meager family larder. My mother shared a bed with her sister, Doris. Her brothers dropped out of high school to take jobs. In contrast, my father was his parents' cherished only son.

Nourished by my grandmother's stories and intrigued by his reticent memory, I tried to imagine my father's Russian childhood for him. The small boy playing hide-and-seek with his sister among bolts of worsted and gabardine in his grandfather's store. The fine china plates piled high with kasha varnishkas, roast chicken and garlic on his grandmother's Sabbath table. The enormous goose-feather puffs that covered him when he went to sleep each night. I imagined his father's trips from Zhitomir to Warsaw on horseback to buy velvet collars and fine woolen fabrics for the women's coats his grandfather sold in his dry-goods store. It did not occur to me that my father might not *want* to remember his early years.

He left Russia three years after the execution of Tsar Nicholas II and his family by the Bolsheviks. In addition to the bloody civil war between the Bolsheviks and the Tsar's White Army, which had claimed thousands of lives all over Russia, western Ukraine had been the scene of some of the worst anti-Semitic violence in Europe since well before the Russian Revolution. Most anti-Semitic pogroms were carried out by Ukrainian nationalist forces and by Cossack horsemen fighting on the side of the Tsar.

In the three years prior to the Steinman family's exodus, there were at least three major pogroms in Zhitomir. "Cossacks!" my grandmother used to hiss, rolling her eyes heavenward with a sense of unspeakable horror.

My father did not remember how he slipped out of Zhitomir at night, with his mother and sister, hidden under straw in an oxcart driven by a Polish farmer. He could not remember what I remember for him: the caresses of his mother, her soft breasts, her hand over his mouth to keep him quiet. He could not remember the itchiness of the straw, the warmth of his sister Ruth's body, the sound of her breath in the dark a counterpoint to the creaking of the cart wheels on the rutted dirt road.

He did not retain these memories, but the loss of them may have been instinctively self-protective. With the good memories, he may have also lost memories of old men laid out on cold cobblestones in the marketplace, wrapped in their prayer shawls, their faces shorn of beards, their tongueless mouths contorted in pain. The four-year-old boy may have been able to forget the dead bloated cows littering the road, the ruined bridges, the ransacked synagogue, the upended tombstones, the bayonet thrust in the belly of a pregnant neighbor, the infant thrown down a well. He may have forgotten the thundering sound of the Cossacks' horses racing through the streets of Zhitomir, a terror his mother would remember until the day she died.

By chance, my father's army regiment had both Russian and Japanese connections. The

Twenty-seventh Infantry Regiment (later part of the Twenty-fifth Infantry Division) was sent to Siberia by the U.S. government in 1918 to join other foreign troops — English, French, Czech, German, Turkish, Greek, French, and Japanese — in bolstering the White Army against the Bolsheviks. It was in Siberia that the regiment earned its nickname, Wolfhounds. After a twenty-five-mile march, the Japanese troops at the head of the column began to fall out along the road. When the United States Twenty-seventh Infantry passed through the scattered Japanese columns, General Otani, the Japanese commander in chief, commented that the Americans marched like Russian wolfhounds. From that day forward the regiment became known as the Twenty-seventh Infantry Wolfhounds. Their insignia shows the profile of the head of a Russian wolfhound with the Latin motto below: "Nec Aspera Terrent," which translates, "Nor do they fear difficult missions."

Though my father displayed little interest in his Russian origins, on some level he apparently still thought of himself as Russian. "I may be a Melancholy Slav," he wrote in one letter home, "but these last two years have made me even more melancholy."

The Twenty-fifth Infantry Division began the year 1944 in New Zealand, an ideal spot for rest and recreation after grueling campaigns on Guadalcanal, New Georgia Island, and Arundel Island in 1942 and 1943. After Guadalcanal, the

Twenty-fifth Infantry Division was known by its nickname, Tropic Lightning. Their insignia was a bright red taro leaf with a streak of yellow lightning inside it.

According to *The 25th Division and World War 2* (the 1946 army-issued yearbook for veterans of the Twenty-fifth), there were "too many distractions" on New Zealand to allow for good training. The yearbook points out that "New Zealand boasted civilized amenities like white women, automobiles, billboards, and traffic cops."

By mid-February 1944, the Twenty-fifth Division packed up and moved out. After two weeks they landed at Noumea, the principal city of the French island of New Caledonia. Here they would train for upcoming combat "somewhere" in the Pacific. (For reasons of security, grunts like Private Steinman were not informed in advance where that combat would be, though there were always rumors.)

The yearbook describes the months of enforced waiting on New Caledonia as "rehearsing the old and learning the new modes and methods of waging war." The exhausted old-timers were relieved to have a long break from the rigors of combat. The newer recruits, like my father, had yet to be tested in the real theater of war. The long wait, the building apprehension, took a toll on their nerves. To keep up morale, there were movies every night. Bob Hope and Jack Benny showed up on New Caledonia's Oua

Tom Airstrip. A few lucky men drew from a lottery a few days at rest camps during the long spring and summer months.

My father's anxiety about impending combat, wherever in the Pacific it was going to be, was compounded by his anxiety about his wife and the impending birth of their first child.

On their last evening together at Camp Fannin, in Texas — just days before he left for the Pacific — my parents conceived my sister, Ruth. Over the next nine months — from January 1944 to September 1944 — while the Twenty-fifth Division was in New Caledonia and New Zealand preparing for combat, Ruth prepared for her own perilous passage. The separation from his pregnant wife exacted an immense strain on my father. September 1, 1944, two weeks before his daughter's birth, he wrote:

Time is purely relative and ordinarily the two weeks lapse due to the crossing of mail from your side of the world to mine never bothered me as long as the mail came in regularly. I just didn't feel that difference of a fortnight or fourteen days. But with the most important event of my life taking place perhaps this very minute, that bridge of time is so very great that every second and minute just keeps pounding away at my heart.

Of course one goes through trying times, terrible strains and ordeals during the course of one's life. But the emotional disturbance of not knowing what is going on with the birth, life and pain and suffering of one's closest, dearest, to one's heart — is the greatest that I have ever gone through.

He had wanted his firstborn to be a girl so he could name her Ruth after his sister. He sent money and specific instructions to his sister-in-law in New York to buy his wife a white gardenia and bring it to her in the maternity hospital. When the cablegram with the good news reached him on September 23, 1944, ten days after his daughter's birth, he was instantly ec-static. "It must be because I so badly want to be with you at this moment and the telegrams never could tell one how you are — I'll never be happy again until I get back to you and Ruth," he con-fessed. He handed out cigars and three cases of beer to his buddies in celebration. "I passed out cigars and the guys all teased me that I wasn't 'man enough' to father a boy. Little did they know how much we wanted a daughter."

For the next three months, his wife entreated him to write their infant daughter a letter. My fa-ther balked. How could he explain the soldier's superstition against writing a farewell letter be-fore combat? How could he make clear how des-perate he was to see a picture of his new daughter?

19 November 1944
And you see Darling — I want to see what

78

Ruthie looks like — then getting Hal Rubin's gift will be lots easier.

In late December 1944, the Tropic Lightning Division was finally ready to move toward combat. They were divided into three groups and boarded ships for a convoy to Luzon. En route they staged a practice landing at Tetere Beach, Guadalcanal. "There were strong cross currents and faulty beach markings," the yearbook reports. Deficiencies in their landing preparations were corrected before the convoy reached its destination of Lingayen Gulf, the Philippines.

Weds, 3 January 1945

Dearest,

By the time you get this letter, the War Department will have released the news of our whereabouts so I can write a little more freely of my thoughts and reactions of a man just before going into combat.

Up until now we weren't allowed to mention that the outfit is going into action or that I'm on a boat but since this letter will be held until our whereabouts are no longer secret, the censorship has been lessened somewhat.

I'm not really as nervous, scared, afraid, or tense as I thought I would be — of course the bullets aren't flying yet — and I'll probably be scared stiff when they start whizzing but right now I'm still perfectly normal and sane.

A whole year of laying around and waiting for this event has perhaps taken the edge off it. When something like that is put off and delayed and drawn out the excitement and expectant thrill dies away — and then — I'm a little too old and staid to get excited at the thought of dangerous adventure.

I'll probably write a few more letters before I leave the boat but there will be a long interval after that before you hear from me again. But you've got to have faith — and remember that "no news is good news." I have the utmost confidence in myself pulling through alright. . . .

Writing has been difficult for me these last two months — with all the preparations for moving really got on one's nerves. I'm sorry if I've written in a vein to hurt your feelings and I'm sorry that I've caused you all the undue anxiety. And it has been difficult writing on the boat — our compartment is so very crowded and unbearably hot. Except at night when I turn in, I stay away from there all the time. The only times I have written were when I've been on Message Center duty at the troops office aboard ship.

Again, I feel physically in the pink — a little heavy but that will be sweated off in no time at all.

I'll write again before I get off this tub. And remember that I think of you constantly — and my love for you will carry me through — Norman

His Russian soul also sustained him through combat. In April 1945, after sleeping on the ground and in holes for over a hundred days during the Balete Pass campaign in Luzon, "living through sights that left an indelible impression" on his mind, he confessed why he believed he had survived:

I've had many a narrow escape, and I have two theories as to why. One is the old Russian adage of "nichevo" — "what the hell attitude" — the other is that someone is looking over me like an angel — I believe it is someone like my sister Ruth and perhaps my little daughter or maybe it's my wife who has so much faith in me.

It was surprising to read my pragmatic father's belief in a talismanic word and a guardian angel. Soldiers have always carried talismans into battle: a lock of a daughter's hair, a rabbit's foot, photos of sweethearts, a family Bible. Pomo Indian tribesmen from California, who fought in the United States Army during World War II, carried special handkerchiefs on which a tribal shaman painted magical geometric patterns. Yoshio Shimizu, and millions of other young Japanese soldiers like him, carried silk flags tucked inside their helmets or worn across their chests. Around their waists they wore *senimbari,* "thousand stitch" belts, which carried the collective good will of their womenfolk.

But my father carried with him *nichevo.* The literal meaning in Russian is "nothing." He carried with him an attitude. Nothing. Zero. Void.

I wrote to my friend Olga, an émigré Russian actress, to ask her what *nichevo* means idiomatically. Olga wrote back, "*Nichevo* means that your father did not care about what was around him. He found something valuable inside him that gave him power to live. Also, *nichevo* means 'OK' attitude, meaning that 'we'll have the end of this nonsense and the day will come and we live normal life.' "

Perhaps the "nichevo attitude" is what the Buddhists call nonattachment. Shrug it off. Concentrate on the breath. It will be over. He would come home. He had *promised* he would come home.

At the United States Holocaust Memorial Museum, I heard an Auschwitz survivor describe the attitude that enabled her to persevere as "the resignation to go on. . . . Okay, God, if that's what you want me to do — I'll do it in order to live." My grandmother used to shrug her shoulders, lift her palms heavenward, and ask rhetorically, "Listen, everything is unbelievable. But what can we do?"

There's a related concept, it turns out, in the Japanese vernacular, the expression *shikata ga nai.* In John Hersey's *Hiroshima,* the first eyewitness account of the aftermath of the atomic bomb blast, a survivor explains: " 'As for the bomb,' she would say, 'It was war and we had to expect it.' And then she would add, *'Shikata ga nai,'* a Japanese expression as common as, and corresponding to, the Russian word *'nichevo':* 'It can't be helped.' "

Shikata ga nai. Nichevo. Nothing to be done but go on. During the Battle of Balete Pass, in Luzon in the spring of 1945, my father came down from the mountains by jeep to Clark Field, near Manila, to pick up supplies for his battalion. Two days later when he returned to his foxhole, it wasn't there anymore. Blasted away by a shell. Was that the spirit of nichevo, the work of a guardian angel, or just damn good luck?

His sister, Ruth, the angel who watched over him, was just fifteen when she died from a heart-valve defect. She had progressively weakened since she was ten or eleven. My grandparents did not exhibit the nichevo attitude when it came to their daughter. They traipsed from specialist to specialist in vain, hoping to find a doctor who could repair the tiny hole in their firstborn's heart. When she died in 1927, my father and his parents never stopped mourning.

Ruth had been my father's best friend and his ally against all the strange experiences of a new land. She broke ground for him, cleared the way. Just as significant, he was her protector. He was quick on his feet and fetched things for her. He reported the neighborhood gossip when she was confined to her bed. Small for his age, he took his role seriously. Ruth was the constant in his life between what was unknown and what was known. Then she was taken away.

Ruth's death was the shadow over my grandparents' lives, my father's life, and, in some way, it was the shadow over our lives, in 1950s Los Angeles, as well. He rarely spoke of her.

In 1951, a year before Jonas Salk discovered his vaccine, my sister, Ruth, contracted polio. She was six. I was just three months old, but Larry remembers the exact day. He remembers when Dad broke the news to our grandmother. The word "polio." A shriek of grief, then weeping. My father reached into the bureau for a container of pills, begged my grandmother, "Take this! Stop crying!"

Norman Steinman locked away deep inside himself those two great sorrows — the death of his sister and whatever had happened to him in combat. These were private sorrows, ones I was not expected to share. I never knew my father to cry.

In the fall of 1945, with combat behind him, my father was able to explain to his wife why he had resisted writing a letter to his infant daughter:

Let me go back about a year ago and describe a scene in New Caledonia. One night Melvin Smith — a Texas boy whom I

had basic training with at Camp Fannin —
came into my tent and we were shooting the
breeze but I could tell there was something
on his mind. Finally before the evening was
over he came out with it. "Steinman," he
said, "would you do something for me?"
"Sure Smitty — shoot," I said, "what is it?"
"Will you keep a letter and some personal
papers for me when we leave the Island —
and mail it to my folks in case I don't come
back?"

He tried to talk the young man out of it. He
tried to cheer him, told him how silly it was to
feel that way. But Melvin Smith insisted. He
died at Umingan on January 29, 1945.

I believe that the fear of dying paralyzed his
will to go on, and that was the cause of his
death. So I had to tell myself every day that
I would be coming home, and when I
started a letter to Ruthie — and I started
many — I just couldn't be glib or jocular or
breezy and once I started to get serious, I
thought of those farewell type letters and
tore it up.

But he didn't tear them all up. He did write
one letter to his infant daughter before he went
into combat. He wrote it on January 4, 1945,
aboard the convoy ship that carried the Twenty-
fifth Infantry Division to Luzon. He finally sent

it home on January 29, the day Melvin Smith was killed at Umingan.

> Pacific Ocean, 4 January 1945,
> Saturday night

Dearest Ruthie,

This is my very first letter to you. I have been very reticent about writing; I can't explain why. Your Mother has been telling you so many stories about me that I don't have to introduce myself, and I fervently hope that when I do come home, I can live up to all of them.

I am writing this letter while sitting on the top berth in a hold of a ship. It is very crowded, cramped, smelly and hot. The sweat just pours off you, whether you sit, write, read or sleep. This is the last letter I will write before we disembark and "Make History" as some bigwig once told us trying to impress us.

Your Mother writes all about you, every detail all around the clock — and I love every word of it. I was a little cross with your Mother when she didn't send the pictures of you at first — she didn't realize that I am getting ready to go into combat and how badly I need to see what you looked like. But I'm sure that she understands now.

I'd like to tell you a little of what you mean to me. You are the fulfillment of a great desire, and a symbol of a beautiful love of two people.

Every man wants a child. It is a fulfillment of his function as a member of society. I especially wanted a daughter — one to take the place of my sister, a wish that I've wanted for some sixteen years. My childhood was very incomplete, and with her passing that void was never filled until you arrived. You are the first of the five that we always planned on having.

I pray that we will be meeting soon — you, Mother and I. Until then, I promise you that I'll always be thinking of you — I won't try any heroics but of course my job and orders come first. I'll be as cautious as humanly possible. I have the Russian attitude of "nichevo" — just Devil may care — and it is a good attitude right now.

As for you — just keep Mother happy and busy so that she won't worry too much during this period of waiting.
I adore you both,
Your Daddy

The convoy reached Lingayen Gulf at 0000 (midnight, military time) on the eleventh of January 1945. When my father wrote this letter to his daughter, he was just days innocent of combat. Ruth was still healthy and whole. Nichevo was still strong enough to sustain him. The enemy was, though just barely, "over there," in a place where Norman Steinman had never been and to which, after the war, he would never return except in memories he either tried to abandon or kept strictly to himself.

CHAPTER FIVE

Speculation

During the month I spent at Fort Worden reading and rereading my father's letters, certain phrases jumped out at me. It was shocking to come across the soldier's blunt, monosyllabic descriptions of his foe: "Those Nips don't give up until they are dead. So we have to kill them all." This language was so alien to the vocabulary of the liberal and tolerant postwar father I thought I knew.

I logged those comments and checked dates. Most of them appeared after January 1945, after the Twenty-fifth Division landed at Lingayen Gulf, the Philippines. From his references to "Hal Rubin's gift," my mother deduced her husband was on the eve of combat, and in one of the few of her letters that was preserved she wrote consolingly, "Being ruthless is a new experience for one as sweet and peace-loving as you."

How does one transform a "sweet and peace-loving" man into a soldier, someone who is expected and willing to kill? Most World War II GIs were civilians hustled from dry goods stores in the Bronx, farms in Tennessee, mines in Colorado, banks in St. Louis. What happened to them when they encountered gruesome combat against the Japanese in the swamps and jungles of the Pacific Islands? What enabled them to kill other human beings? And, just as important, what psychological scars did they bear after they returned home?

These questions haunted me. Hoping to find some answers, I raided the shelves of the history section of the tiny Port Townsend library. When I returned to Los Angeles, the questions returned with me.

In his book *On Killing: The Psychological Cost of Learning to Kill in War and Society*, Dave Grossman, a psychologist and army colonel, focuses on the long-term effects that the experience of killing exacts on the soldier's psyche. Along with other military historians, Grossman believes the heaviest burden of war is usually carried by army infantrymen — men like my father.

He cites one particular World War II study: After sixty days of continuous combat, 98 percent of all surviving soldiers suffer some kind of psychological damage. I remembered how, in one of his letters, my father complained, "Our division seems determined to set a record for consecutive days of combat on the front lines." By the time the campaign for Balete Pass was over, the Twenty-fifth Division had been committed to the front lines for 165 days of *continuous combat*.

By far the most startling World War II statistic I read in his book was that only 15 to 20 percent of army riflemen in World War II would fire at the enemy. They did not run or hide, but they *simply would not fire.* To the question, Why did these men fail to fire? Grossman explains that there is within most men an intense resistance toward killing their fellow man. He then describes the techniques the military uses to overcome this innate and powerful reluctance. They must inculcate the idea that one's enemy is not a human being.

"For the war to be prosecuted at all," writes historian and World War II vet Paul Fussell, "the enemy of course had to be severely dehumanized." When someone is dehumanized they no longer have a face, a family, a history, a reason to be alive, or a reason to allow them to be left alive. "When you see a dead Nip, you won't care. But no matter how many times you see a dead Yank, you'll never get over it," a seasoned soldier told journalist Murray Kempton when he first landed on New Guinea.

This was true on both sides. John Dower points out in his landmark study *War without Mercy: Race and Power in the Pacific War* that this dehumanization contributed to the brutality and mercilessness of the conflict in the Pacific. "As World War II recedes in time it is easy to forget the visceral emotions and sheer race hate that gripped virtually all participants in the war," Dower writes, explaining how "each side portrayed the other as its polar opposite: as darkness opposed to its own radiant light."

"Bestial apes" is how Admiral William F. Halsey referred to the Japanese. "Kill Japs, kill Japs, kill more Japs," he exhorted the troops. American wartime propaganda posters depicted the Japanese as subhuman and repulsive, "louseous Japanicas," vicious jungle creatures, tailless apes to be exterminated.

On the other side, Japanese soldiers were told they were on a divine mission, fighting against a demonic foe, that American GIs were monsters who rifled corpses for gold teeth and took no prisoners alive. The Americans and British were considered savages who "ate raw meat and had mouths dripping with blood." Roosevelt and Churchill were depicted in Japanese political cartoons as debauched ogres. The Japanese military turned the war itself — and eventually the concept of mass death — into an act of collective purification: "One hundred million people, one mind" was a popular slogan during the war.

By the 1930s, the traditional Japanese warrior code of honor called *bushido,* which called for humane, courteous, and kind behavior (adhered to by the Japanese Army in World War I), had been radically altered by the Japanese government and military, who inflamed feelings of hatred toward the enemy. The military training endured by Japanese draftees, often boys from poor farming communities, was a system of rigorous discipline that included beatings, psychological humiliation, and exhausting physical exertion. Among veterans, the slang for new recruits was *issen gorrin*, Japanese for the sum of one sen, five ren (less than one penny) — the cost of their draft postcard. Military training was deliberately designed to prepare the recruits to brutalize others. I learned that historians refer to this system of indoctrination as "socialization for death."

Senjinkun, the military manual that all Japanese soldiers were supposed to obey in World War II, made several principles absolutely clear. One was obedience to one's superiors, who were considered representatives of the emperor himself, the highest moral authority. Another was that being taken prisoner by the enemy was a profound disgrace to the emperor, to one's family, to one's village, to the entire nation. Suicide was preferable to surrender. *Gyokusai*, the word means "to shatter like jewels," was the phrase for an honorable death in lieu of surrender. To GIs like my father, this fact alone made the enemy seem inhuman. You approached a Japanese soldier warily, even if he was waving a white flag. He might pull out a grenade and blow himself up — taking you with him. To the Americans, the Japanese seemed to want to die, to glorify death. My father's statement — "Those Nips don't give up so we have to kill them all" — grimly sums up the prevailing attitude among American infantrymen toward their enemies during the Pacific War.

★ ★ ★

After their landing in Lingayen Gulf in January, the Twenty-seventh Infantry Regiment fought a fierce battle in the flat fields around the town of Umingan, which lasted until February 4. After that, they pushed inland over steep forested terrain toward the strategic Balete Pass in the Caraballo Mountains, where the troops of General Tomoyuki Yamashita, commander of the Japanese Fourteenth Area Army in the Philippines, were entrenched in the hills.

The men in the Twenty-seventh made the arduous climb in fierce heat through dense jungle, often tripping over thick vines and sliding off trails where monsoons had eroded whole chunks of mountainside. Five months of fierce fighting passed before the Americans could claim victory over Balete Pass. What close calls had my father been through?

The first mention of the Japanese flag came in a letter on February 13, 1945, after Umingan was captured and they'd begun the ascent up Highway 5 toward Balete Pass: "I have a Japanese flag now. My first thought was to send it to Hal Rubin, but then, I decided that I'll probably sell it to some Marine for about fifty dollars. So I'll hang on to it awhile."

The envelope containing only the flag (no note) was postmarked March 3, 1945. Over the next several months, while the battle raged around him, my father apologized to my mother for sending it home: On April 24 he wrote, "I'm

94

so very sorry that I sent you the Jap flag. It was a little boy use of bad judgment. I'll never send any more such gruesome souvenirs home. I promise." In June, after the battle was over, he fretted, "Don't put the flag on display. I should have sold it to some rear echelon glory hunters." On July 1, a full four months after he'd mailed the offensive article, he was still suffering over it: "It was an adolescent impulse that will only be rectified when I am home with you and have apologized personally." Four days later, July 5: "Your letter today mentioned how upset Mrs. R was about George's Purple Heart. Well, we all make mistakes. George is sorry that he ever mentioned it. Just like I was when I sent the Nip flag home. All George got was a scratch on his wrist from a piece of shrapnel and the medics put him in for it."

Norman Steinman regretted the distress he had caused his wife when she opened the envelope and confronted the flag and what it possibly meant. But I wondered if there might be another explanation why he had such a difficult time forgiving himself for sending the flag home.

In his essay "On Moral Pain," writer-philosopher Peter Marin describes the psychological damage done to a man when he must balance the *obligation* to kill with the *guilt* that results from fulfilling that obligation. As Marin points out, it's a tragic catch-22: "The soldier is damned if he does, and damned if he doesn't."

My father had violated his own standards of

morality by picking up a war souvenir, and it troubled him deeply. He had done what soldiers have always done, taking what they have conquered.

Japanese flags were a common souvenir for many American soldiers. "We used to say that the Japanese fought the war for their emperor, the British for glory, the Americans for souvenirs," wrote historian William Manchester. Souvenir is from the Latin *subvenire*, to come up again, to come to mind. Many of the men who took flags from the battlefield would later find, like my father, that they did not want the stories provoked by those old souvenirs to "come to mind." Yet they couldn't bear to destroy them, either. That would betray their memories of their dead friends, their own grief and anger.

Thousands of years of human warfare have made clear that men can be permanently damaged by their "temporary" transformation into killers, by months of constant shelling and bombardment. In the American Civil War, this damage was called "soldier's heart"; in the Great War, soldiers who were "shell-shocked" were taken to a hospital where doctors zapped them with electrical current, insisted they renounce their symptoms and return to the front. In World War II, it was called "combat fatigue" and it was not uncommon, though the Pentagon brass insisted there was no such phenomenon, that anyone who claimed to suffer from it was a weakling or a malingerer. In 1943, in Sicily,

General George S. Patton slapped and kicked a decorated soldier hospitalized with shell-shock and called him a "yellow bastard."

After Vietnam, the phenomenon entered the psychiatric lexicon as "post-traumatic stress disorder," which journalist David Harris, who was imprisoned for draft resistance during the Vietnam War, has perceptively defined as "undigested grief."

For men who returned home from World War II, repression was the standard medical prescription. "Time will heal," doctors told those men who thought to ask for help. The men who fought the brutal war in the Pacific — who'd seen their buddies ripped apart by Japanese bayonets, who'd filled their nostrils with the stench of death — buried their anguish. In refusing to speak of it, they might succeed in holding the horrors at bay.

For Norman Steinman, all those years of never crying, never venting his sorrow, trying to restrain his rage, to suppress the nightmares — all those years of placating his "soldier's heart" must have clogged his arteries with grief. He couldn't tell his wife the very worst that happened. He could send her the flag, but he couldn't tell her how he got it.

My innately gentle father and his buddies *allowed* themselves to believe that the enemy they fought in the jungle was subhuman. How else could they have tossed white phosphorus bombs into caves where there were living men? How else could the Japanese have tortured and beheaded civilians, prisoners of war, unless they believed likewise? In contrast, once I knew that my father's enemy *had* a name, was *indeed* a human being, he *became* human. Those simple words, "To Yoshio Shimizu," brought a shade to life. I was not just in possession of a flag. I was in possession of a *name*. That name belonged to a person with a family and a history.

Though I trolled through his correspondence for a definitive answer, my father's letters never described how he actually acquired the flag. I tried to imagine the battlefield meeting between my father and Yoshio Shimizu. My imagination balked at the image of my father killing someone.

In March of 1945, Private Steinman wrote of leaving the battlefield during combat in a jeep with two other Jewish GIs — Sam Wengrow and Morrie Franklin — for Passover seder at Clark Field. Taking a cue from the 23rd Psalm, which we'd recited at both my parents' funerals, I mentally prepared a table in the presence of my father's enemy. I constructed an unlikely scenario. What if my father and his buddies encountered Yoshio Shimizu on the way to the seder? What if it happened, say, like this: My father is in the jeep with his buddies Morrie Franklin and Sam Wengrow. They have an overnight pass. It's two and a half hours over bumpy terrain to Clark Field. They navigate sheer drops more than thirty-five hundred feet, hairpin turns. After forty grueling minutes, my father says to Walter, the driver, "Can you stop here? Gotta take a leak."

"No problem," says Walter and he stops the jeep.

While my father pees, Sam Wengrow ventures farther into the brush. Out of the bushes appears a ragged Japanese soldier, waving a white flag. The man is jabbering. Sam points his rifle at the man. He could be booby-trapped, dangerous. He keeps babbling, follows the trajectory of Sam's rifle and marches to the jeep.

"Look what I found," says Sam to his buddies. My father takes some communication wire and ties the prisoner's hands behind his back. "I'll sit in the back with him," he tells Sam and off they go. My father has his carbine pointed at the man's side. They'll throw him in the stockade at Clark.

The man is terrified, relieved, famished. Shaking like Jell-O. My father gives him a piece of salami from his own private stash; he gives him a cigarette. The Japanese soldier wolfs the salami down. Who knows what they'll do with him, the prisoner must be thinking. He's still alive. He might as well eat.

"Tokyo boom boom boom?" Sam says to the prisoner over his shoulder from the front seat. Does he know Tokyo is being bombarded with incendiary bombs? The man shakes his head, he doesn't understand. The rhythm of the bumpy road makes him drowsy. He falls asleep with his head on my father's shoulder. "You've got a new friend, Steinman," Morrie teases.

They arrive at the seder with the dozing prisoner. Inside, the chaplain is holding up a matzoh and the assembled are reading responsively: "Behold this is the bread of affliction our forefathers ate in the land of Egypt. Let all who are hungry enter and eat thereof. Let all in who want to observe the Passover. This year here, next year in Jerusalem. This year as subjects, next year as free men."

The front door of the mess hall has been left open for the prophet Elijah, as is customary at a seder. There is even an extra wineglass on the table. On the "Amen!" Norm, Sam, and Morrie escort Yoshio Shimizu inside. The wine has just been blessed, is now being poured. The officers look askance at this breach of protocol. "They brought a *shkutz*," says a captain, and the men all laugh. My father seats Yoshio beside him at the table and unties his hands. He grabs the Manischewitz and pours him a glass. The wine is sweet like plum wine. It is Passover; you're supposed to recline at the table. You're supposed to drink four glasses of wine instead of one. These are mnemonic devices to help us remember the significance of the story of Exodus told on this holiday.

The seder plate is passed around. There is a bare bone and a burnt egg to symbolize the burnt offering Moses made to God on Mount Sinai. The tradition is for the youngest son to ask the ritual Four Questions. But there are no children here, so nineteen-year-old Private Cohen from Schenectady is drafted for the job. "Why is this night different from all other nights?" How was this war different from all other wars? The men pray they'll never invade the mainland, that God's secret weapon will spare them for next year in Jerusalem. The men chant "Dayenu," meaning "It would have been enough." It would have been enough if the Red Sea had parted, it would have been enough if Moses' staff turned into a snake. It would have been enough if God had spared the firstborn of the Hebrews. They drink more sweet wine. They sing *Chad Gadya*, that children's song:

> Then, the Angel of Death came
> And slew the butcher
> who killed the ox
> that drank the water
> that quenched the fire
> that burned the stick . . .

All the men are high by now, even Yoshio Shimizu, who pounds out the rhythm on the table with a Navy spoon. My father is in such a jovial mood, he even sings that Russian song with all the "heys."

After the last cup of wine is drained, Yoshio Shimizu rises from the table and faces my father. He presses his good-luck banner, a silk flag, into Norm Steinman's hands, bows deeply, and is led away.

★ ★ ★

Most probably, it did not happen like that. A letter my father wrote in the Communications tent while a hard rain fell realistically depicts his attitudes toward Japanese POWs.

25 June 1945

The roads are really a sea of mud. When we take the Message Center run via jeep, I always get covered from head to toe with mud. People talk about the Pony Express Riders in our history — but I don't think any of those guys had any more thrills or dangers than our twelve-mile ride daily. But as I've said before, it can't go on forever. This paper is getting a little damp from the rain, but it will still be legible I hope.

Just got a call, that they are bringing a Nip prisoner in — if it isn't too dark out I'll take a picture of the little bastard.

I've written a letter to Mom care of your address. Trying to time it with her arrival. You'll have to write all her reactions with Ruthie.

Time out. Prisoner just arrived. The usual crowd of hanger-oners sweating him out. I did take his picture — the bastard is scurvy looking. We told him to sit down and he squats or kneels — like he was praying to Shinto. Don't know why I keep writing about the prisoner. Now the son of a — is staring at me while I'm writing. He probably

102

thinks we'll kill him. He does look scared.

Oh well — this is all in a day's routine. I'll write more tomorrow. So I can get this off in today's mail.

Perhaps the flag was simply abandoned. After Umingan, my father describes a battlefield strewn with objects the Japanese soldiers left behind: "The Nips must have cleared out in such a hurry that they didn't wait to take anything with them. Last night I slept on a Jap blanket and used a real pillow. George even had a mattress. We were all envious."

Or, perhaps it happened like this: my father kneeled over the cold body of a young Japanese soldier who had fallen in front of his eyes in the fierce fighting around Balete Pass. In the yearbook of the Twenty-fifth Infantry Division and World War II, published just after the war, there's a description of Japanese dead "littering a battle-torn hill." Perhaps my father noticed a scrap of silk still clinging to the lining of the dead soldier's helmet, and plucked it out. Perhaps, in the dizzying heat, he folded that banner carefully and placed it in his pocket. It didn't weigh anything.

CHAPTER SIX

The Gift

It was a powerful impulse to imagine my father's enemy as a real person. Of course, my life was not threatened by grenades or snipers. I had the luxury of speculating who Yoshio Shimizu was, what he might have felt, where he came from. I wanted to know if, like his enemy, Yoshio Shimizu had a young child he'd never seen. Did he have brothers, sisters? Did he come from a big city? A small village? Had he suspected that the emperor was not a god but a man? Had he somehow survived the war? Was he a grouchy executive who'd lived in Nagoya all these years? Was he a shopkeeper in Gifu, tormented by nightmares? Had he been a foot soldier or a commander? Had he beheaded POWs in Bataan? Huddled in a foxhole sharing stories about home?

As I imagined Yoshio in more detail, and as I read more about the history and ethics of the conflict, I contemplated what form might best express what I was learning about the war. For many years, creating a performance or dance/theater piece had been the way I gave order to my investigations.

I could create a performance piece or a one-act play about the imagined battlefield meeting between my father and Yoshio Shimizu. I could use images from my father's letters, both real and imagined: the American GIs drunk at the seder with the Japanese POW; the two soldiers singing themselves to sleep at night in their fox-holes; a meeting on the battlefield at night against a projected film clip of the emperor riding his white horse; scenes of my father parting from his young wife; and Yoshio Shimizu, reluctant to go to war, receiving his good-luck flag from his family in Japan.

Inspired, I applied to a foundation in Japan to create this dramatization of the two soldiers and the lost flag. Their rejection was swift and disappointing. It also turned out to be a gift in disguise.

The foundation had misinterpreted my project proposal to mean that I would actually perform *with* the flag. A program officer there took it upon himself to explain why this would be a bad idea:

If the Japanese audience realized that the flag was not in the possession of its original owner, presumed dead, they would find this repugnant. Should you return the flag, in fact, to the family of Yoshio Shimizu, it is my opinion that your efforts would bring a lasting reward to your soul — the supreme

105

act of reconciliation between an American soldier and a Japanese soldier as carried out by the posterity of the conquering nation.

The program officer's suggestion lit flares in my mind: What if what began as artistic speculation could instead become a physical gesture in the real world? What if it were possible to actually find Yoshio Shimizu or his family and what if I could *actually* return the flag to them?

I had no clue how to begin locating a person connected to some fifty-year-old smudges of ink on a piece of Japanese silk. I tried the Japanese Consulate in Los Angeles, with no success. I was open to suggestions.

A friend who spoke Japanese came up with the address of an organization in Tokyo that sounded quite helpful: the Japanese War-Bereaved Families Association. If I wrote to them, she suggested, surely they would help me find the family of Yoshio Shimizu. I wrote immediately.

Months passed. No word from Tokyo. It was late 1994, and the fiftieth anniversary of the end of World War II was just half a year away. In the United States, as in Japan, there was considerable debate about how to commemorate this momentous anniversary. The argument about how to portray the dropping of the first atomic bomb was spilling across the Pacific, and igniting incendiary emotions. The politics of memory between the two sides of the Pacific War were deeply conflicted.

In the United States, the controversy centered on the Smithsonian's proposed exhibition about the *Enola Gay* (the plane that dropped the bomb on Hiroshima), with veterans groups accusing the museum of revisionism and historians accusing Congress of pandering to veterans.

In Japan, the loudest controversy centered on whether or not the government should issue an apology for Japan's brutal actions in Asia during World War II. ("A small dry cough of remorse," is how *New York Times* correspondent Nicholas Kristof termed the government statement that was finally issued.) The newspapers were filled with new accounts of the Korean comfort women forced by the Japanese military to provide sex for Japanese soldiers during the war.

The Japanese War-Bereaved Families Association, I later learned, was one of Japan's most influential nationalist organizations, a potent lobby that was putting its muscle behind the fight to block a war apology in the Japanese Parliament. Although opinion polls showed that the great majority of Japanese was in favor of an apology, the association supported the outrageous claim that Japan had fought "a war of liberation" to free Asians from the yoke of Western rule, and that to admit otherwise would dishonor the Japanese war dead.

If I had known that, I could have guessed their response to my query. Whatever the association discerned were my motives (at the time not exactly clear to me), they wanted no part of my search. They declined without offering any specific reasons.

One Sunday, while reading readers' queries in the *New York Times*, one question made me sit up and take notice: "How do I find the grave of a British soldier from World War I who is buried in a military cemetery near London?" Hmmm. I scribbled my own query to the *New York Times* Question Man: "I would like to find the record of a Japanese soldier who fought in the Philippines in World War II," I wrote. "I found his good-luck banner in my father's mementos and would like to return it to the family."

Several weeks later, the phone rang and I picked it up to hear a deep warm voice: "I'm Paul Freireich from the *New York Times* and I'm going to take on your question," he informed me. "Tell me everything you know."

Within weeks, Mr. Freireich had located and communicated with a Mr. Chitaru Satake in the Office of Records Research in the Social Welfare and War Victims Relief Bureau in the Japanese Ministry of Health and Welfare. Mr. Satake had agreed to open an official search through Japanese government documents to find Yoshio Shimizu or his survivors.

I sent Mr. Satake a photograph of the flag and a letter explaining what I knew about when and where the banner was found. I thanked him in advance for his efforts, and then I waited.

★ ★ ★

One grant did come through that spring, a modest stipend from the local arts commission to conduct storytelling workshops for recent immigrants, especially those who lived in neighborhoods hardest hit by recent urban unrest. Teaching these workshops brought me no closer to Japan, but by learning to listen more carefully, I began to see how seemingly disparate stories can bring people together in unexpected ways.

For my first session, four participants showed up. There was Mark, a blind Cambodian; Naz, from Soviet Georgia; Wendy, a Chinese student; and Lucy Mendez, from El Salvador. As an exercise, I asked them to talk about gifts they had received, something that helped them remember the person who gave them the gift.

There were blank stares. Okay, an example. I showed them my wedding ring, the one that my father had bought for my mother when she was just nineteen, the antique gold band formed of five Cupids linked head to toe. "There are five Cupids," I said, "because my father wanted to have five children. When I see this ring on my hand, I think of my mother and father."

Lucy suddenly spoke up. "I have a gift from my father. He died in the civil war in our village. I have a lock of his hair," she said, fingering her own. Naz's father had been killed by a stray shell two months earlier in the ethnic strife in Azerbajian. He'd been a journalist for the daily newspaper in their town. All his life he had wanted to come to America. Naz kept her father's papers and his visa in a black wallet in her purse. Mark rustled in his pocket and pulled out a tiny brass Buddha. His eyes filled with tears. An amulet from his mother, a victim of the Khmer Rouge.

In that humble classroom I contacted a world much larger than my own, a world in which a parent's death at sixty-one from a sniper's bullet or execution squad — rather than at seventy-four from a heart attack — was not so uncommon.

The word *bereaved* comes from the Anglo-Saxon word for "robbed." Someone or something you love is snatched away from you. By a pirate, a rogue heart, a firing squad. Until I discovered my father's letters, I hadn't realized that the war had stolen him away before I was born.

The people in my workshop had all suffered great losses. Even if their own children never learned the specifics — how Naz's mortally wounded father slumped over in the street in front of his newspaper office, or how Lucy's dad was buried in a mass grave of headless corpses behind their village, or how Mark's mother was carefully photographed by her torturers before she was executed — their lives would reverberate with the loss of their parents in ways their parents might never have imagined. They would become part of their dream life, their heritage — the way my father's experiences in the mountains of northern Luzon were part of mine, though he had never spoken of them.

Part of my heritage is a gift I received from my Russian grandmother. She managed to bring with her from Ukraine an exquisite set of ceremonial silver wine cups, each incised with the spires and rooftops of the Jewish quarter of Zhitomir. Three of the five were kept in a glass hutch in my parents' condo, and were stolen in a robbery four months before my grandmother died. The theft of these family valuables — the loss of this slender link to the past — demoralized my entire family.

I sometimes take one of the remaining silver cups that my grandmother bequeathed to me from my top bureau drawer. I close my fingers around it; it fits snugly in the palm of my hand. This cup traveled with my father, my aunt, and my grandmother through the maelstrom of a civil war. Yet what, really, are the family valuables? The silver cup I've admired so many times would mean little to me without my grandmother's stories. The silver spires etched on its surface would be merely the generic outlines of a town somewhere in the Old Country, not the complicated terrain inhabited by loyal in-laws, gossiping cousins, a tender grandfather. The Japanese flag would be the generic banner of an enemy army if I did not possess the name of its owner, who, like my father, was no doubt dreaming of his family through many a long night on Luzon. The name on the flag was the key to Yoshio Shimizu's history, his place and his time.

CHAPTER SEVEN

Questions

Six months later, the letter from Mr. Chitaru Satake finally arrived. I ripped it open with trembling hands and stared at the incomprehensible Japanese script — trying to will it into meaning. I could not wait another minute to find out what it said. Hurrying out to the street, I searched for pedestrians with Asian faces. Seeing none, I scanned the storefronts on either side of the post office: Gap, Pottery Barn, J. Crew. I glanced inside a Banana Republic and rushed up to a young Japanese American clerk. "Me? Read Japanese? No way!" she said in a Valley Girl accent.

A banner hanging outside a Japanese restaurant caught my eye. I ran inside the sushi bar clutching my precious letter. "Can I help you?" asked the manager. Could she read Japanese? I asked. No, but the sushi chef did. After wiping his cleaver on his apron, he translated the letter on the spot. The search for the family of the soldier looked "promising," wrote Mr. Satake, "but there is more research to be done. Do not be disappointed," he cautioned me. "Sometimes, in cases such as these, the families do not wish to be contacted." The sushi chef handed the letter back and, without ceremony, resumed gutting his mackerel.

To help facilitate direct communication with the ministry, a friend, who had lived in Japan, referred me to a young woman in Tokyo named Amy Morita. She took a personal interest in the flag, perhaps because of her own complex family history. Amy grew up in the Philippines after the war, when anti-Japanese sentiment was quite strong. Her grandmother was a Japanese American woman who married a Japanese national and moved to Japan before the war. In Japan, Amy's grandparents were arrested several times by the military government for being "American sympathizers." On the other hand, across the Pacific, her grandmother's Japanese American family members were interned by the U.S. government. "I believe that war is full of tragic irony," Amy wrote to me, "and the stories I heard during my childhood have given me the opportunity to think about the war and many of the sad dramas created by it."

The weeks passed. There was still no definitive word about the family. Perhaps they belonged to the Japanese War-Bereaved Families Association and would find my request distasteful. Amy had explained to me that the process used by Mr. Satake's office was painstaking. Records from World War II were handwritten. Shimizu was a common name, so other identification — primarily the names of those who had signed the flag — must be confirmed. I imagined a huge roomful of clerks in a gray government building dutifully sifting through numberless boxes of yellowing documents, and thousands of Shimizus all over Japan receiving a solicitous call about some crazy woman in America bent on returning a flag to their family.

Through my new job at the downtown library, I met a large community of writers. A Filipina novelist invited me to a reading of her new novel. Cecilia and I had talked about my father's letters from the Philippines, my desire to better understand his war experiences, the flag, my hopes of returning it. Her book was based on her parents' experiences as *guerrilleros*, fighting the Japanese in the mountains of northern Luzon during the war.

The reading was scheduled in a hole-in-the-wall bookstore in a minimall called Luzon Plaza. I drove by the mall every day on my way to work, and had never once considered stopping, though the word *Luzon* flashing in red neon always brought to mind my father and the war.

Entering the little bookstore was like stepping into another world. The people there, most of them Filipino American, switched from Tagalog to English and welcomed me warmly.

Before Cecilia began, the bookstore manager announced, "Afterwards we will all eat together. We've brought Filipino food." My stomach flip-flopped at the thought.

Even though my father never named the specific source of his aversion to Asian food, it was so dramatic that I intuited the reality. I even came to believe it had been passed on to me genetically. I'd read about Filipino delicacies like *balut* (unhatched duck embryos), pigs' ears, skewered chicken intestines. To mention the Philippines at all in my father's presence was to elicit a grunt of disapproval and discomfort.

On the trays were lovely buns with bean paste, spicy chicken empanadas. "Spanish and Asian, our two culinary influences," the bookstore manager said. After the reading, I made chitchat and then sidled up cautiously next to the tray. I picked up a golden pastry and, thinking no one was looking, sniffed at it gingerly. Cecilia silently appeared at my side. She'd been observing me. "You know," she began with a smile, "if you really want to understand your father's experience in the war, you should go to the Philippines."

The Philippines was not a country I'd ever had any desire to visit. Reading my father's letters had only reinforced my antipathy: "No matter what I look at in the Philippines, be it a rice paddy, stream, or hill or dale it reminds me of something sad and bitter. Through my eyes I can't enjoy anything this island on the Pacific has to offer. It's always associated with the boys who will never come back."

Nevertheless I knew immediately that Cecilia

was right. I nodded as my teeth bit down on the flaky bun to the salty, slightly sweet taste inside. It wasn't bad.

That night I decided to ask Lloyd if he intended to accompany me on the trip to Japan.

It was my obsession to return the flag, not his. Why should he go on a trip that was bound to have its share of awkward and uncomfortable moments? Though he was passionate in his own life and work about the need to build cultural bridges, his feelings about the Japanese were conflicted. Thirteen years older than I, he remembered wartime blackouts in Los Angeles. Among his first drawings was a cartoon of Hitler, Mussolini, and Hirohito behind prison bars, kamikaze planes on fire. As a child, he'd been exposed to the prevalent American war propaganda and had internalized the resentment most Americans felt toward Japanese during the war. Those feelings lay there, unexamined, alongside his more humane impulses.

I was pleased when he decided, on his own, that he would go. I wanted his support, but I wanted it freely given. I was also relieved. I liked to think I could make the trip alone, but having my husband as a travel partner gave me more courage.

"Then, what would you think about going to the Philippines as well?" I asked, though I wasn't exactly sure just what we would do there.

"We'll go to Balete Pass!" he answered without hesitation. "We'll find the marker on the battlefield where Norman was in combat." Of course! It was obvious that was what we would do. We'd rent a car in the mountain city of Baguio, and drive up to Balete Pass ourselves. It sounded entirely plausible.

There was still no word from Tokyo. The disastrous earthquake in Kobe dominated the nightly news, filling me with foreboding. Just a year earlier, the disastrous Northridge quake had flung us from our bed onto the floor. I'd seen firsthand the devastation an earthquake could wreak. I had no idea where in Japan the Shimizus lived. What if they lived in Kobe? As my nighttime worries amplified, I began to question my entire venture. What was driving this obsession to find this family?

Others questioned my obsession as well.

Through an informal network of friends and relatives, I'd located three Pacific War vets in the L.A. area: Peter Lomenzo, a retired Arco executive; Baldwin Eckel, a retired high school physics and math teacher; and Sylvan Katz, a retired administrative judge. They had all seen combat in the same area of the Philippines as my father had.

Peter had been a lieutenant with the Twenty-seventh Infantry Wolfhounds, my father's regiment, from Pearl Harbor through the occupation of Japan. He'd been a battalion commander in the battle for Umingan, and a staff officer in the battle for Balete Pass. Baldwin, who grew up in Japan, was a missionary's son, and learned Japanese as a child. He worked in Army Intelligence interrogating Japanese POWs in Luzon. "I wasn't a typical American soldier," he told me. "I was an American who grew up in Japan, as a Japanese, with all of the stresses, joys, and sorrows of that experience." Baldwin had even interrogated General Yamashita after the surrender. Sylvan served with the army's Thirty-second Red Arrow Division, which had engaged in fierce combat with Japanese troops on the rugged Villa Verde trail in Luzon.

Each of them was, in varying degrees, skeptical of my impending mission to return the flag. But they all responded supportively to my desire to understand what they had been through, and all three agreed to meet with me.

I interviewed each of them. Over the subsequent years, these three men continued to share their often painful stories and feelings with me. I'd phone Sylvan or Peter if I had questions about military terms or protocol, the logistics of the infantry, the geography of northern Luzon. Baldwin, with his profound grasp of Japanese language and culture, could answer questions about words like *shakata ga ni,* or explain the Japanese code of *bushido.*

Our exchange filled a gap on both sides. For me, it was a vital opportunity to ask questions I'd never been able to ask my father. For these men, it was an opportunity to tell stories they'd yet to reveal to their wives or children.

I first visited Peter Lomenzo just months after his wife of fifty years had passed away. He showed me a picture of a radiant young woman: "This is the place where I met Marie on the docks in New Zealand. Three girls came over to ask for dates to go for a dance, and I picked Marie." Marie, a native New Zealander, had been one of those "distractions" the army command had been worried about when they moved the Twenty-fifth Division from New Zealand to New Caledonia for training. Together, Peter and Marie had raised a family of nine children.

I noticed a samurai sword on the mantel. "My grandson is interested in that," Peter commented. "He asked me, 'Can I have that sword, Grandpa?' I said, 'No, that's from Japan. It's very sharp and heavy. I keep it up there. I can't get it down for you.'" He paused, smiled slightly. "He said, 'Well, can I have it when you're dead?'"

After my first visit with Baldwin Eckel, he followed up with a letter. Opening up to me about the war was not without emotional hazard:

I must confess that I have a hard time with "war stories." My defense has been to ignore the whole mess, though I must admit you were the first person to whom I was able to relax and tell things about myself that I never was able to do with others.

About a week ago, I was roasting a ham for some family friends. I was cutting a

119

plastic wrapper off the whole ham when the knife slipped and cut my wrist. It was a cut over a wound I had from the war on my right arm. When I looked at my wrist, I had an uncontrollable urge to scream. I kept my mouth shut, finished my task, even though my wife who was standing next to me offered to dress the wound. I refused and took care of it myself. That night I had an awful dream, waking up thinking about a foolish thing I did that could have, really should have killed me. It is these kinds of flashbacks that worry me.

Sylvan Katz's resentment toward the Japanese was still evident, though he was focused on works of good will — bettering the lives of the Igorots, Filipino highlanders with whom he'd made close ties during the Luzon Campaign. These tribal peoples had carried mail to the troops, helped ferry out the wounded on stretchers. Sylvan personally maintained a scholarship fund to send the children and grandchildren of these Filipinos to college. He spoke animatedly about his protégés, and told me about the extent of the brutality the Japanese exhibited toward their enemies as well as the civilians of the countries they occupied during World War II. He sent me articles clipped from magazines, copies of interviews with Filipino villagers, and a videotape of the infamous Unit 731 of the Japanese Imperial Army, who airdropped fleas carrying bubonic plague on random Chinese villages and subjected men, women, and children to vile medical experiments worthy of anything Mengele dreamed up at Auschwitz. In a note accompanying the videotape, Sylvan wrote, "These images are gruesome, but I know you do want to know the truth."

During one conversation at Sylvan's comfortable apartment in Santa Monica, we took a break after an hour and a half of talking. As I walked down the hallway to the bathroom, I noticed a framed Japanese flag, just like the one I'd discovered with my father's letters. This one was in pristine condition. The Japanese calligraphy on it was even more elegant than on Yoshio Shimizu's flag. When I returned to the couch beside him I gently asked, "So, Sylvan . . . what about the flag?" The judge's handsome face grew instantly somber. The apartment was very quiet except for the ticking of the clock. Sun streamed through the bay windows. We sat in silence for several moments.

"I will *not* talk about it," he said. "And I do *not* plan to return it." He paused before adding, "What's more, your father is probably turning over in his grave right now." I could hear the pain in this good man's throat, the warning to pry no further. More secrets. I had zeroed in on a wound. Sylvan had zeroed in on my own naivete.

Days later my brother Larry phoned and asked, "Would you be returning this flag if it were a German flag with a swastika on it?"

He had a point. Having grown up in a Jewish household where unnamed relatives had perished in the Holocaust, I wonder if I could have seen past that symbol to whatever humanness might have existed on "the other side."

For many who had been caught in the maw of the Pacific War — American vets, Japanese citizens bitter about their country's legacy of militarism, certainly many Koreans and Chinese who had suffered Japan's barbaric occupation of their countries — the Rising Sun flag was just as loaded. In 1987, Shoichi Chibana, a grocer in Yomitan, Okinawa, was arrested for tearing down and burning a red sun flag at the opening ceremony of a national athletic meet. At his trial, Chibana argued that many Japanese on Okinawa still considered the flag a "loathsome symbol" of wartime militarism and sacrifice. In 1945, the Japanese Army had ordered the mass suicide of eighty-two Yomitan civilians as a gesture of loyalty to the emperor. My desire to return the flag, or the flag's desire to be returned, was turning out to be more morally complicated than I'd bargained for.

When I arrived at my office the next morning after an agitated and sleepless night, I stared with disbelief at a fax on my desk from Amy Morita. The Ministry had located Hiroshi Shimizu, the younger sister of the soldier. Yoshio had died in the war, but his sister lived in the town of Suibara near the city of Niigata, on the northwest coast of Japan.

The Ministry had provided Amy with an address, but no phone number. Weeks passed without further word. Then Amy called from Tokyo around midnight. She had spoken to Hiroshi Shimizu. She had simply searched through the phone directory for Niigata Prefecture until she found the number.

She was thrilled with her detective work but sounded one major note of caution: "She sounds old and is rather confused about your visit," Amy said over the crackling phone line. The morning after Amy's call, I bought two round-trip tickets and nailed down my leave of absence from work.

I busied myself with travel details, like finding the right container for the flag. I wasn't exactly sure what "right" meant. Not too big, not too small. Not flimsy, not cute. Dignified. Finally, in a fancy stationery boutique at the Beverly Center Mall, I saw what I wanted — an austere, flat, navy blue leather box, which contained very expensive Crane's stationery. "Could I just buy the box?" I inquired hopefully. The clerk raised her eyebrows. I remembered suddenly that cranes are revered in Japan, and bought the box without further hesitation. I was, after all, alert to omens.

On the way home, my car drove itself to the cemetery. Not until I turned off the ignition did I fully realize where I was. I walked into the mausoleum, and sat on a stool in front of my parents' crypt. I stared at the silent wall, at the incised

words on the bronze plaque: NORMAN STEIN-
MAN: A JUST MAN.

I tried to guess what my father would think of
this mission, this obsession of mine. I was about
to fly halfway around the world to give this flag
to the sister of his enemy. Was I doing the right
thing? I was planning to visit Balete Pass, the
place he considered hell on earth.

28 March 1945, The Philippines

Dearest,
The days are really telling on everyone here.
All the eighteen-year-old youngsters have
suddenly begun to look years older. And
many a gray hair has been added to my
noggin.

This outfit has been overseas since Pearl
Harbor, and every man here is bitter. They
have been through every campaign from
Guadalcanal on. And right now it seems
that our division is striving to set a new
record for the most consecutive days in
combat on the front lines. I know I sound
bitter, but those are the conditions. And I'm
at the stage where I don't give a damn.
We're all tired and suffering from combat
fatigue. But I would probably still have the
same sentiments even if I were well rested.

I'm still physically well — and a good soldier always gripes. So don't worry about me.
I really haven't changed from the guy you
know. Just a little harder and tougher to get

along with. But I do love you — Norman

Was Sylvan Katz right? I couldn't help wondering. Was my father angry, restless in his grave?

PART II

Japan

CHAPTER EIGHT

Bombs under Tokyo

On April 7, 1995, fifty-one years after my father crossed the equator on his way to war, I was crossing the Pacific for the first time, gazing out at clouds and water through the windows of a wide-body jet en route to Japan. In my backpack under my seat was the box containing the Japanese flag on which was written the name of my father's wartime enemy. Beside me, my husband dozed peacefully, a magazine open on his lap.

I reclined my seat, closed my eyes, and tried to relax. For weeks, months now, I'd imagined possible scenarios of the moment when I would hand over the flag. I screened them now in my mind. In one version the American woman walks alone at dusk across a rice paddy, a mysterious pack on her back. The sky is blood red. Black clouds descend like swooping dragons. The woman knocks on the door of a small thatched hut in the middle of a deserted field. The door creaks open; a frail, stooped woman peers out. The American tries to speak to her but the old woman shakes her head. She closes the door, pushes the visitor away. Second version: The old woman lets the visitor come inside, opens the box, then faints when she sees the rust-colored speckles on the flag. In yet another, I'm standing alone in the town square of some remote Japanese village, clutching my box while curious villagers eye me from behind half-drawn curtains.

By July of 1945, my father assumed he was going to see Japan for the first time as part of a massive Allied invasion of the Japanese islands. He was dreading it.

The invasion of Kyushu, the southernmost of Japan's home isles, was scheduled to launch on November 1. Half a million American soldiers, sailors, and airmen were to assault the island's southern beaches, backed by an armada of three thousand ships, including twenty-two battleships, and more than sixty aircraft carriers.

It was the weary combat troops in the Pacific, including the Twenty-seventh Regiment, who were slated for the Kyushu invasion. My father was deeply depressed about the planned campaign and the obstacles still to be surmounted before he could come home safe and sound. "Maybe I ought to turn psycho," he confessed. "That won't be too hard. I'm pretty far gone already."

In the summer of 1945, Peter Lomenzo was a twenty-seven-year-old army battalion commander with the Twenty-fifth Infantry Division on Luzon. He vividly recalled the briefing session he attended for the Kyushu invasion:

Several hundred of us — Army, Navy, and Marines — were in a heavily secured gymnasium, on little folding chairs, like little card table chairs. They had these big photographs of the landing beaches in Japan. My battalion had a spot on one of those damned beaches. I knew it. And it was awful. Our first objective was to be a heavily fortified military air strip a short distance from the beach. You can imagine the kind of support around a military base. I'd been worried and scared before, but this was the first time I was really frightened. Was I up to leading 1,000 combat infantry men ashore?

All they kept talking about was the medical support. I thought, "We're all going to get killed." There were more medical units involved in the landings than anything else. It was going to be bigger than D-Day. Hundreds of thousands of troops. And we were going to be in those early landing waves.

There was good reason for Peter Lomenzo and Norman Steinman and all of the American infantry forces to dread a campaign on the Japanese mainland. The U.S. military expected the Japanese would be prepared, their beach defenses fortified with several hundred thousand soldiers and perhaps five thousand aircraft. Kamikaze pilots would dive-bomb the ships at anchorage. Japanese soldiers would pilot huge torpedoes, called *kaiten,* into American ships. The coast of Kyushu was studded with caves, and the mountains there were more rugged than Okinawa's. Japanese civilians were prepared to fight to the death rather than dishonor their country. Mass suicide was not an unlikely scenario.

After the news reached Luzon of the atomic bombing of Hiroshima *and* the entry of the Russians into the war against the Japanese, rumors of an imminent Japanese surrender circulated among the infantry. Infected with a new optimism, my father wrote on August 9:

> I'll start right in with the greatest news broadcast of my countrymen the Russians declaring war. That news was more exciting to us here than the VE broadcast. Why maybe now I can see my chances for getting home are a reality — and Lordy, I hope that it isn't necessary to have an invasion. The Russians and the atomic bomb should be the combination to cause the Japs to surrender without losing their ugly face.

On August 11, the Twenty-fifth Division received the first report from San Francisco that the Japanese had accepted the Potsdam Ultimatum (in which the United States, Britain, and

China announced the terms of a surrender) with the reservation that the emperor be allowed to keep his white horse, a phrase that sounds as if it were lifted from a fairy tale rather than from a sober political document.

Peter Lomenzo recalls how, on August 12, in the midst of a deadly serious discourse by a senior officer on the landing beaches for the invasion, "an officer walked briskly down the middle aisle up to the platform and said, 'Men! I want your attention! The President has just announced the unconditional surrender of Japan.'

"The entire gang erupted in sheer joy and disbelief that anything like this could just up and happen. We did thank GOD."

After all the tense anticipation, there would be no invasion of the Japanese mainland. The doggies on Luzon went wild. As my father reported: "From the Colonel down to the Privates — the boys in town really rioted — just helping themselves to all the liquor available. I detailed a cook to get up and serve coffee all night long. What a night."

Drunken revelry continued around the clock. The beer held out for days on end. "We can't seem to get back down to earth," he wrote, also reminding his wife that when he finally got home, he would need "rest, plenty of rehabilitation. I always thought that term a great joke but it's true. What is really the matter is that I can't enjoy anything and the key to the answer is you. Also, it will take a long time if ever to forget the horrible things I've seen."

I couldn't feel the plane's movement through the air. It felt as though it were simply suspended in space. I thought of my father suspended in anticipation, waiting thirty-five days off the shore of Nagoya on a "Navy tub" called the USS *Natrona*.

By September 24, 1945, his regiment had boarded troop ships in Lingayen Gulf in the Philippines bound for Japan. Instead of invading the mainland in what he and his buddies feared would be a bloody nightmare, the Americans were about to join their fellow servicemen as the victorious and occupying army.

> We're on the same type of boat that we left New Caledonia to hit this beach but the situation is so very different now. There isn't the tense feeling and the fear of going into combat for the first time and the thought that many amongst us wouldn't come out of it. Now, not only do we know our destination but we know that no lead or shells or bombs will be thrown at us — and everything is clear sailing. Also, all the reports did state that not one soldier has been hurt in the occupation of Japan so far.

Nevertheless, the prospect of mingling with their all-too-recent enemies did not please the troops.

6 October 1945, USS *Natrona*

We are all annoyed at the idea that we have to be nice to the Nips. We would like to do to them as they did whenever they took over a city or country. The Nips will think us crazy for not doing what they would do under similar conditions. Why, we may even lose face.

Anyway we're getting a unit of fire for our weapons before going ashore. I feel better already, I thought for a minute that we would just go in with empty rifles. But there is no chance of anything happening. The Nips are playing it smart. They're really taking us for suckers, I do believe.

What am I getting mad about? The war is over — aren't we supposed to kiss and make up?

In the weeks of waiting on the ship, the men watched *I Married an Angel* with Nelson Eddy and Jeanette MacDonald in the mess hall; they spent hours playing cards: "Insipid games like pinochle and we make the games so very important trying to concentrate on the playing and time goes by that way. Then we read anything we can get our hands on — magazines so very old, all kinds of trite fiction anything just to kill time and try to forget the rolling of the ship."

There was constant friction on board between army doggies and navy men:

135

21 October 1945, USS *Natrona*

We were disturbed by the officers who just came in for a shakedown inspection. It seems that the boys have been taking the Navy's spoons and forks from the mess hall for their personal possession and now the Navy is complaining and wants them back.

A Navy spoon is always an infantry doggie's prize possession. A spoon next to one's rifle is the most useful instrument of war. I own a Navy spoon that I got from the USS *Oxford* — the ship we hit the beach of Luzon on — but I wouldn't give it up for the world. I intend to keep that as a souvenir of the campaign.

My father turned thirty on October 14, 1945. The army postal service came through, delivering to the tub nine letters from home (three from his parents in Los Angeles, six letters from his wife in Brooklyn), two pipes, and pictures of his little girl at her first birthday party.

This is my third birthday in the army. The one that I'll never forget and cherish in my memories always, is the first one, when my Dearest arrived in Texas before I shipped out, the best present a man could ask for. I was the happiest soldier alive. The second one spent in loneliness in New Caledonia, wondering if I'd ever see you again, and the third one just marking time aboard a Navy transport and dreaming of coming home to you and Ruthie and being together for all our birthdays.

The ship was abuzz with rumors, including one (false) that they'd have to go ashore without their weapons. No soldier who'd faced the Japanese infantry in the jungles of Luzon was happy about that.

15 October 1945, USS *Natrona*
One of our boys who has been ashore told me of the strange reaction he had when he first saw the Nips. Some of them are still in uniform roaming the streets. He said, "I saw some that looked like those I shot at!" and some that looked like those he'd hit. He just hates the bastards hates them all — and he couldn't stomach the sightseeing and dumb sailors who acted like they were on a joy cruise in a port. It was interesting listening to him because I've often wondered how I'd react.

On the day Lloyd and I arrived in Tokyo, the cherry trees were in bloom, the dollar had plummeted relative to the yen to the lowest point since World War II, and everyone was anxious about toxic nerve gas. The city was on high alert. Just a few weeks earlier, on March 20, the shadowy sect Aum Shinrikyo had released sarin nerve gas in the Tokyo subway, killing twelve people and injuring fifty-five hundred. In what one Cabinet minister described as "a war" between the sect and the Japanese government, citizens of one of the world's safest countries grappled with unaccustomed fear whenever they took subways or went to public places. Members of the cult and their enigmatic blind guru, Shoko Asahara, had not yet been apprehended.

For our first two days in Tokyo, we stayed at the house of an American acquaintance whose husband was the Tokyo correspondent for network television. Marjorie's home was extremely comfortable, lavish by Japanese standards: two stories, four bedrooms, three baths. With the devalued dollar, the network paid an unfathomable twenty-four thousand dollars a month rent on the house. In the local shops, Marjorie showed me the hundred-dollar cantaloupes, beef at fifty dollars a kilo. A large pizza cost seventy-five dollars.

That spring was also the twentieth anniversary of the fall of Saigon, and Marjorie's husband was on assignment in Vietnam. Marjorie had her hands full taking care of two young children, ten and two, in a foreign city.

I quickly became friends with ten-year-old Laura, a wise, dreamy child with long brown hair and an infectious grin. She went to an elite international school in Tokyo and, like most kids in Japan, she was assigned hours of homework each night, an expectation that generated ongoing friction with her mother. Laura preferred to spend time making collages out of Japanese wrapping paper, creating imaginary stories with her dolls and stuffed animals, or drawing in her sketchbook.

Lloyd and I were offered the baby's nursery for a bedroom. We fell asleep quickly that first night, exhausted from travel and time changes. I woke in the predawn, jet-lagged and dream-drunk. I dreamed I'd come to Japan to find the Japanese pilot who'd dropped my father, alive and naked, over the Pacific Ocean.

It was a stunning fall, in slow motion as falls in dreams often are. There was the shock of seeing my father's pale flesh against the brilliant blue sky. He had a slight paunch and his black hair was gray, as it was at the end of his life. And he was falling, his legs tumbling over his head and then around again . . . what was the expression on his face? In the dream, I tried to see — but I couldn't.

I lay still in the half-dark. My father did not die in the Pacific, I told myself. He came home, he raised a family with my mother. He ran a pharmacy. He cracked corny jokes. He wanted me to go to law school.

I rolled over next to Lloyd. His skin was clammy and hot. He was burning with fever, the onset of a nasty flu. I opened my eyes, disoriented. Humpty Dumpty leered in the half-light. The toddler's rocking horse was an emperor's ghostly white stallion.

I pulled on a robe and tiptoed down the hallway to the kitchen to make tea, to try and clear my head. Marjorie was already in the kitchen, herself jangled awake by a nightmare. "There were Asian men planting landmines all over the house," she whispered loudly. "One of them was crouched over the kitchen sink."

All over Tokyo — maybe all over Japan — an epidemic of nightmares had broken out. The horror of the subway gassings had people in its grip. No wonder Marjorie was nervous; some of Laura's schoolmates narrowly missed being on the subway train that had been gassed a month earlier.

A groggy Laura appeared at the kitchen door as we stared into our tea. It was Saturday, no school. "What's the plan?" she asked.

Marjorie was adamant that we should not take the subway anywhere. When Aum Shinrikyo members vacated their compound, they took their bags of sarin nerve gas with them. "CNN reports say they're planning a kamikaze attack on a big crowd of people," Marjorie said. She'd been up late watching the news and her eyes were red.

Laura stirred her hot chocolate. "What's a kamikaze?"

"Like terrorist bombers," her mother explained, "like in Israel where they do a suicide bomb into a crowd of Jews."

"Oh," said Laura, alarmed. "I don't think I'll go outside at all."

"No, you'll survive," her mother insisted.

140

★ ★ ★

I piled thick blankets on Lloyd, tried to make him comfortable with hot tea and aspirin. Getting sick at the beginning of our adventure was not part of the plan. What could I do to make him feel better? He insisted I go out without him. Marjorie was a wreck from lack of sleep and the baby was fussy, so Laura and I set out on foot together for Meiji Shrine, the largest Shinto temple in Tokyo.

We wound our way through the maze of streets toward Meiji. The Jingumae neighborhood was designed in medieval times to deliberately confuse any enemy who might approach the shrine. We emerged on the main boulevard into the thick of consumer culture: We passed a Gap store, Banana Republic, a Benneton boutique, Kentucky Fried Chicken, McDonald's, a billboard for Kirin beer featuring a grinning Harrison Ford.

We reached the Outer Gardens of Meiji Shrine, and entered under the huge tori gates. I'd read that on October 21, 1943, this was the place where thousands of drafted students from Japan's colleges and universities gathered for the biggest public send-off of the war. Thirty-five thousand young men stood at attention with rifles on their shoulders, facing bleachers filled with sixty-five thousand people. A cold rain fell, and for three hours the new recruits were bombarded with patriotic rhetoric, which was also broadcast to the nation. A new recruit named

141

Shinshiro Ebashi, who until his induction was a student at the elite Tokyo Imperial University, set the tone with his speech: "We, of course, do not expect to come back alive as we take up guns and bayonets to embark on our glorious mission of crushing the stubborn enemy." Prime Minister Tojo also addressed them: "The decisive moment has come when one hundred million of us take up battle positions and overcome the hardships confronting our fatherland."

Tojo reminded the new soldiers that the United States and Great Britain were also sending their students to war. "But I do not have a shred of doubt that you will overwhelm them in spirit and in combat capability." After the rally, the recruits marched through the streets of Tokyo to the plaza facing the Imperial Palace, where they shouted "Banzai!" for the emperor.

I thought about those young men standing out in the rain as we walked down the long pebbled pathway toward the shrine. Laura was walking with her eyes focused intently downward. I grabbed her arm just before she collided with someone coming the opposite direction.

"Be careful," I entreated her.

"Looking for acorns," she muttered.

It began to rain lightly. I insisted Laura open her red umbrella. She could not have cared less about getting wet. She was determined to continue her search through the pebbles for an acorn. Suddenly, she let out a squeal. Among the numberless stones, she'd found a real prize:

a tiny carving of a squirrel. I was dumbfounded. She was ecstatic.

"It's like finding a needle in a haystack!" I exclaimed. Laura didn't know the aphorism. "Well," I said, "It's so improbable. What are the odds? A million to one? That you'd find a carved squirrel among all these pebbles? Not a million to one, a billion to one."

"Or," Laura said, squinting her eyes, "what are the odds that you would find that flag?"

Her skillful segue took me aback. "Well, after my father died, I needed to go through his things."

"Well, what are the chances you would even look for it down in that storage locker?" she said. "In fact, what were the chances your father would even survive a war?"

She knew she didn't need to wait for a reply. "Not very good," she said. "Not very good at all."

CHAPTER NINE

Shrine of the Peaceful Country

On the ninth of September 1945 — a week after the Japanese had signed surrender papers aboard the USS *Missouri* — the commanding officer of the Twenty-fifth Division was officially notified of the division's mission during the occupation of Japan: to disarm the Japanese and see that they stayed disarmed.

As the division yearbook understates, "Lack of information on the exact nature of the occupation made planning difficult." Inventory and disposal teams were responsible for destroying Japan's war-making capabilities. There were thousands of tons of war matériel to be destroyed and disposed of, thousands of miles of roads to be covered in reconnaissance. Men from the Tropic Lightning Division were to provide guards for the trainloads of Koreans — forced laborers in Japan during the war — en route to embarkation ports on the island of Kyushu.

On October 19, 1945, after five weeks of cramped confinement on the USS *Natrona*, the

Twenty-fifth Division finally disembarked in Nagoya. The city, the size of Detroit with a prewar population of 1,350,000, had been almost completely destroyed by American bombs. As he walked the ruined streets, my father wondered how a country "so poor and backwards dared to wage war against the United States."

The son of a coat merchant, he noticed right away that peoples' clothes were shabby, that no one wore good leather shoes, just shoddy wooden clogs or sneakers. Women dressed in baggy pants made of coarse cloth. "Only the comfort girls wear kimonos all the time — that's how the fellows can spot the houses of ill repute," he wrote home.

Like most Americans, my father knew no Japanese personally. He knew little, if anything, about Japanese culture. Japanese films were unknown in America, Japanese literature largely untranslated. Not until 1953 was there a major exhibition of Japanese art in the United States. At the time of Pearl Harbor, Japan was as mysterious for most Americans as it had been when Commodore Perry sailed into Tokyo Bay in 1853. What my father knew about the Japanese he'd absorbed from wartime propaganda, or learned from bitter combat. Now he strolled among a stunned populace whose sons and brothers and fathers, until just recently, he had been determined to kill and who had been equally as determined to kill him. (In fact, the home of the Japanese Twenty-sixth Infantry —

145

which had opposed the Twenty-fifth Division on Guadalcanal in the early stages of the war — was located right outside Nagoya.) My father's first reactions were predictably tense:

> 19 October 1945
> The first Nip I saw I had a strange feeling, watching him walk unconcernedly and unmolested. I felt like squeezing off my trigger — all my reflexes of wanting to kill the SOB came into the fore. Then after a while, I saw so many of them that I got over the feeling. Before long, as we walked along, the kids started yelling "hello," "choo gum," "cigarettes?"

A few days later, he walked past a boys' elementary school, commenting in despair:

> They were all lined up in the courtyard and some Tojo-looking bastard was addressing them. They were in military formation, and when he finished they all snapped to attention by command and rendered the hand salute — and so on. All the kids in schools wear some kind of uniform. I'm beginning to think that we'll never stamp out militarism in Nipland.

The sullen resentment on the faces of middle-age men, the women's smiles, the cheerful greetings of the children must have elicited a peculiar set of emotions. In his letters, he never admits to feeling he is in any danger, though he mentions an expedition by jeep with his buddies to a distant village, where it occurred to them that the inhabitants "may not even know yet that the war is over."

After a few weeks, his letters take on a more positive tone. He noted that after the Japanese realized "we're not going to hurt them in any way" they seemed "sincerely happy to have us here." They were "very polite and outwardly friendly — most cooperative, no trouble at all." They were industrious workers and meticulously clean. "Sometimes I think even their custom of removing their shoes to enter their homes is a good one," he conceded.

His biggest thrill came from the spectacle of the Twenty-fifth Division engineers collecting and destroying Japanese military equipment. "Our Cannon Company Boys are towing the Nip planes and then the tractors roll over them — then the flame throwers burn them up — I feel as gleeful seeing this happen as the Nazis did when they burned books."

On his rambles through Gifu, the former resort town twenty miles north of Nagoya, where the Twenty-fifth Division eventually established a garrison, he kept his eye out for souvenirs to bring home, but none met his standards. "Most of the trading is for kimonos — but although one can get them for about ten packs of cigarettes, I haven't seen any that I would be proud of. They are all made of sleazy rayon, commonly known as *shmate* — but most of the boys were grabbing anything they could get."

There was one thing, however, that caught his attention. High on the shelf on the second floor of a bombed-out department store in Gifu was a doll — an emperor on a white horse. He wanted it for his daughter. Before he could reach for it, another soldier grabbed it.

Lloyd was too ill for sight-seeing. We'd moved to a hotel to spare Marjorie and her children from the flu and to ensure maximum quiet for sick bay. I prayed he'd recover by the time we were supposed to leave for Suibara, where Yoshio Shimizu's family lived. I left him sleeping fitfully in a darkened room with Tylenol and cold green tea at his reach and then I set off to explore Tokyo on my own.

I'd heard enough speculation about Asahara's minions and their cargo of sarin gas to convince me to stay off the subways. It was a beautiful spring day in Tokyo anyway, and I was glad to be aboveground. My destination was Yasukuni Shrine, where Japanese honor their war dead. My map indicated that I could get there by walking through the Imperial Gardens surrounding the emperor's palace.

It was lunch time as I navigated through the crowds of suited salarymen, garrulous schoolgirls in thigh-high pleated skirts, elegant women wearing pastel spring ensembles in delicate shades of coral, topaz, seafoam green.

Friends who'd been to Tokyo told me not to miss the bustling fish market in early morning, the antique district, the fifties rock 'n' rollers at Harajuku. But I was irresistibly drawn to Yasukuni Shrine. It was a place that always came up in discussions of how Japan dealt with its wartime past.

"Meet me at Yasukuni," was the traditional parting phrase that Japanese Imperial soldiers gave one another as they went into combat. In wartime Japan, the highest honor a soldier could look forward to was for his spirit to be enshrined at Yasukuni, a place where the emperor himself came to worship and pay respect.

I reached the Outer Gardens of the Imperial Palace, one of the few open spaces in the center of crowded Tokyo. Behind its graceful turrets and ancient stone walls lie the official residences of the emperor and his family. In the late nineteenth and early twentieth century, a passenger on a tram passing by the palace was expected to rise from his seat and bow to the emperor. The palace itself was a focus of almost mystical veneration during the war years. When Emperor Hirohito announced the surrender on August 15, some of his more fanatical Imperial Army officers performed ceremonial suicide in front of the palace enclave. (Several hundred of his exhausted and grateful subjects also gathered to cheer the news of war's end.)

The government established the imperial cult

of State Shintoism in the late nineteenth century, at the time of the great government reform called the Meiji Restoration. Japan was then emerging from a feudal system into that of a nation-state. The absolute authority of the emperor, up to that time a powerless figurehead, was seen as a way to unify the country.

State Shinto encompassed the beliefs that the emperor was God, the direct descendent from the Sun Goddess Amaterasu. The emperor was perceived as a father, and thus the people were annointed with Divine Power. Orders from a superior — in the government, in the army, at school — must be obeyed without question.

Before that, the Japanese freely mixed religious philosophies — Buddhism for funerals, Shintoism for weddings. Shinto was practiced primarily as a folk religion. People worshiped the divine in the forces of nature. A big rock, a rice paddy, a stream could all contain a spirit. Buddhism wasn't appropriate for a state religion because it was an import from China. Shinto, by contrast, was homegrown.

By the early 1930s, Japan had become a military autocracy. Military drill was part of the regular curriculum in elementary schools. In 1931, the Japanese took over Manchuria in China, and established the puppet state of Manchukuo. In the increasing number of armed conflicts that ensued, as the "Buzz Saw of War" destroyed more families by consuming husbands and sons and fathers, the military became like a surrogate family with the emperor as the nation's great patriarch.

After 1936, any citizen who even dared to look at the God/emperor was subject to arrest by the police. After Pearl Harbor, the emperor was practically immured behind the walls of the Imperial Palace; he rarely ventured outside the grounds. The Japanese military wanted an emperor who was both distant and yet at the same time, awe-inspiring.

It was no coincidence that most photographs of Hirohito show him on horseback. From the lofty haunches of his magnificent white stallion named Shiroyuki (White Snow), the five foot three inch emperor was impressively regal. On the ground, he looked like a frumpy businessman.

In his surrender speech on August 15, 1945, the emperor addressed his subjects for the first time. In what has been termed "one of the great understatements in the history of politics," the emperor told his subjects, "The war situation has developed not necessarily to Japan's advantage, while the general trends of the world have all turned against her interest." The emperor asked his people "to bear the unbearable and endure the unendurable."

By virtually all accounts the radio reception was terrible, and to the millions of his subjects who anxiously gathered to hear his message, it was difficult to understand what was being said. Nonetheless, what was shockingly clear was that the emperor himself was speaking. He spoke with a human voice. From the battlefields of Luzon to the border between Russia and China on the Eastern Front, when battle-hardened soldiers were informed that the emperor had surrendered, many wept.

Walking through the gracious East Gardens of the Imperial Palace, what I sensed in the design of the landscape and distant palatial rooftops was remoteness. The current emperor was somewhere over there, across the moat that separated the impenetrable palace walls from the public park.

Visitors to the park were involved in their own private activities. Young lovers embraced on benches, an old man dozed in the sun, tourists flashed Fujis and Nikons, taking portraits of one another against the scenery of gingko trees and well-tended cedars. Some older women, wrinkled faces framed by odd white bonnets, dutifully raked leaves.

It was in the emperor's name that young soldiers climbed into torpedoes packed with three thousand pounds of explosives and were launched underwater toward American submarines and certain death. It was in the emperor's name that Japanese soldiers on Luzon placed grenades on their stomachs, pulled the pins, and blew themselves up.

The emperor cult was abolished by order of the Allies after their victory in 1945, a confusing reversal for many Japanese. What had been preached as official dogma was, after August 1945, prohibited as dangerous military propaganda. Ironically, it was the American government, on General MacArthur's advice, that decided to keep Hirohito on the throne, albeit not as a deity, and to shield him from retribution. MacArthur felt he needed the emperor and the military bureaucracy in order to rule "indirectly," to rally citizen support and prevent civil unrest in a shattered society. A handful of military officers were tried and executed for war crimes by the Allies, but the emperor himself was exonerated and his war responsibility denied and ignored. Most scholars agree that this decision by the Allies may have forever clouded the subject of Japan's war guilt. If the emperor, in whose name all barbarism had been committed for twenty years, was not guilty, then who was?

"Where is the emperor?" wartime Prime Minister General Hideki Tojo asked from Death Row shortly before he was hanged as a war criminal. Even during his long lingering illness, which led to his death in 1989, Emperor Hirohito never issued any statement admitting direct responsibility for his role in the war.

I walked underneath a massive metal torii gate — as tall as an eight-story building — and stepped onto a grand tree-lined promenade leading to Yasukuni. My shoes made a peculiar sound as I walked on the innumerable smooth pebbles.

A flea market sprawled informally on the outskirts of the park grounds. The vendors sipped tea and traded gossip. Along with pottery, kimonos, and old quilts, there were several samurai swords on lacquer pedestals, and a Nazi armband displayed atop a military trunk. The aroma of octopus pancakes wafted from an open-air lunch counter, nearly derailing me from my intended course. I continued on past the huge wooden portals of the Outer Gate, with its golden sixteen-petal chrysanthemum — the divine seal of the emperor — mounted far above my head. The shrine itself was a modest wooden structure, its interior off-limits to all but the attending Shinto priests and the families of the war dead. People stopped in front of it, tossed a few coins in the slatted wooden repository, clapped their hands in the Shinto custom, and made their wish or prayer.

The inner grounds of Yasukuni Shrine were bathed in the translucent glow of pale pink cherry blossoms so revered by the young kamikaze pilots as symbols of the evanescence of life. Under the boughs, a number of older men wearing white armbands hosted an outdoor exhibit, mainly crude paintings of kamikaze pilots about to depart on their last, glorious missions. About six thousand Japanese, ages eighteen to thirty, died in suicide attacks in the war, many during its final weeks, some even after the surrender.

Yasukuni Jinja (which translates as "Shrine of the Peaceful Country") was established in 1869

154

by order of the imperial government, and dedicated to "the celebration and consolation of the spirits of all those who died to defend the emperor and the empire." It was intended at its inception to honor loyalists who died in the Meiji Restoration, but as time went on, it included imperial subjects who died in later wars. Some 2,450,000 Japanese war dead are enshrined as "guardian gods," or *kami,* at Yasukuni Shrine.

Here at Yasukuni, Yoshio Shimizu would be considered a deity.

In 1946, the occupation government demoted Yasukuni from a state shrine to a private religious shrine. But there are many among the powerful right-wing factions in the government who would like to see its former status reinstated.

Yasukuni is still controversial in Japan today, a focal point for nationalist patriotic sentiment. Every August the country waits to see whether the prime minister will make the traditional visit to Yasukuni. In 1994, though Prime Minister Murayama declined to make the visit, a renegade group of his Cabinet ministers defied a high court ruling by openly worshiping here.

In the Yashukan, the war museum adjacent to Yasukuni, I appeared to be the only non-Japanese person in the exhibit hall. Yasukuni and Yashukan are meant for Japanese visitors, not Americans. Most of the explanatory text was in Japanese, and I considered asking someone to translate for me. But the other visitors appeared to be deeply immersed in their own private experience, and I decided not to intrude.

One eerie aspect of Yasukuni is that the World War II exhibits are not shown in the context of a disastrous militarism that brought death and misery to millions of Japanese and others. To the contrary, even photographs of Prime Minister Tojo and General Yamashita, both executed as war criminals, are accorded honor here. At Yasukuni, you almost feel as if Japan won the war.

There is a War-Dead Memorial Peace Prayer Hall proposed for a site adjacent to Yasukuni by the Japan War-Bereaved Association, which publicly contends that Japan did not engage in "aggressive war." The continuing debate over the meaning of the project illustrates the gulf that splits Japanese society on the issue of war responsibility. Its contents are as contentiously debated in Japan as was the Smithsonian exhibit in the United States on the dropping of the atomic bomb. As the Irish peace scholar Terence Duffy has pointed out, "Arguments concerning the assumed 'title' of the facility are central to the controversy, since it is not clear whether the project is conceived as a 'war' or as a 'peace' museum."

Yashukan covers several eras of Japanese militarism, including the feudal Tokugawa period, when Japan was divided into warring shogunates. I walked into a hall displaying samurai armor. Mournful *shakuhachi* flute music wafted from a boom box in a corner. Helmets, lacquered red inside, some improbably tall, were augmented with gilded metal horns or horsehair plumes, or fanciful crests representing snowstorms, catfish tails, lightning bolts. Metal face masks grimaced from their pedestals. Whole suits of armor wired together — ridged and riveted breast protectors, leggings, hinged forearm plates — formed rigid, glowering homunculi. The fearsome personae of the warriors who once wore this empty armor were still palpable. The peach-faced kamikaze pilots, whose memorabilia filled the adjacent rooms, must have looked back to this military tradition with great pride.

The English-language brochure states that the aim of the museum is to pray for the repose of soldiers' souls "and for eternal world peace," but the darker, unmentioned stories that are also integral to the events commemorated at Yushukan came to mind. When I looked at the certificate recognizing "the brave actions of the 13th Flight Squadron in Nanjing (formerly Nanking), China in December 1937," my thoughts turned to the Nanking Massacre — a six-week orgy of terror in which the Imperial Army ran amok, bayoneting babies, gang-raping women by the tens of thousands, summarily executing military prisoners. When I stood in front of the shiny black steam locomotive in the courtyard, which, the sign proclaimed, "holds the distinction of being the first to pass the junction at the opening of the Thai-Burma Railway," I thought about the starved and tortured British and Canadian prisoners of war who laid the tracks.

It's not that I expected to see in a Japanese military museum a memorial to the Korean comfort women, the Chinese victims of Unit 731, or the American GIs who died on the Bataan Death March, but those outrages were, to my mind, ever present.

For a *New York Times* article, correspondent Nicholas Kristof asked a Shinto priest at Yasukuni what the requirements were for becoming a god. What about soldiers who had committed atrocities — raped Chinese women or tortured POWs? "I did not get a clear answer," he reported, "but as far as I could tell, any military person, no matter how brutal, became a *kami* upon death in combat."

Where I found poignancy in Yasukuni was not, however, where it was intended — in those spectacular displays like the gorgeous color panorama of the Divine Thunderbolt Corps in "final attack mode" at Okinawa. Instead, I gravitated to the glass cases that contained the humble personal effects of the war dead. Here was the human face of war: notebooks, binoculars, a small rocking horse, a harmonica, reading glasses, a torn photo of a child, a protractor and compass, a cloth doll. Kamikaze soldiers, elegant in their long white scarves, smiled from sepia photographs. I looked at a glove, a belt buckle, a toothbrush, a spoon.

In one case there was a flag like the one I

would soon return to the sister of Yoshio Shimizu — the same blood or rust spots, and holes in the silk. I examined one of the museum's most famous displays, a poem written in human blood on a rice paper scroll, which was exhibited in front of a gleaming seppuku dagger: last words, not translated into English, from a soldier who committed ritual suicide. I looked up from the glass case in revulsion. I glanced out a window that opened out toward an ordinary apartment building. On the landing, someone's laundry was drying, their umbrellas and bicycles stashed away. I felt restored by these everyday objects, by the fact that this room of the dead looked out on the living.

Tired by hours in the museum, I decided to take the train back to the hotel. As I waited on the platform, I recalled my father's letter about a crowded train in Nagoya during the occupation:

> 1 November 1945
> Since we are the conquerors, we just walked on the station platform without buying tickets and boarded the trains first. Soon the Nip populace began filing in — and although I am a conqueror — I couldn't stand to see Nip women with infants slung on their backs papoose-style standing while I sat. So I got up to give them my seat and they kept bowing and smiling and thanking me over and over again. Wonder if the Nips ever did that in places that they occupied?

159

Individual acts of kindness came naturally to my father, though every incident that happened to him in Japan was filtered through the lens of his anger and bitterness toward the Japanese military, his sorrow over lost friends.

22 October 1945, USS *Natrona*
Just happened to think of a charming letter my friend received from his sister-in-law. She thanked him for all the boys that did the fighting and helped bring Peace to the world, and she mentioned some of his friends who were wounded and she thanked him for safeguarding the security of the world so that her son won't have to participate in a war in his generation. Well, I hope that is true.

But we over here — the combat veterans — feel that the only real heroes are those that gave their lives in the supreme sacrifice and those unfortunate ones who were maimed for life physically or mentally.

The train was very crowded, and according to the map, I needed to make a change after two stations. I somehow managed to get lost. "Sumimasen. Excuse me. Do you speak English?" I asked a young student wearing a severe black military-style school uniform with a high collar and brass buttons. His hair was cropped short, the slight beginning of a mustache showed above his lips, which parted into a shy smile. "Chicago? You know Chicago?" he inquired with enthusiasm. "I was on homestay in Illinois." He insisted on escorting me all the way to Akasaka Station, near the hotel.

If, fifty years ago, this young man had received a red envelope summoning him to war, would he have gone? Undoubtedly yes. The Japanese writer Kenzaburō Ōe writes about how, every day in his school during his childhood in a remote corner of Japan, the teacher would ask the students one by one, "What would you do if the Emperor called upon you to die?" "I would take a knife and rip open my belly," the child was obliged to reply.

I returned to our room just as Lloyd woke up from fevered sleep. I stretched out beside him on the bed that filled most of our tiny room, alternately feeding him and slurping ramen noodles from a cardboard cup that I had bought from a 7-Eleven around the corner.

After looking at bullet-pierced, blood-stained military uniforms at Yasukuni, I was ready for some escape. I turned on the TV. The English language channel featured *Gone With the Wind*. As I dozed off, Scarlett and Rhett fled General Sherman's army against a flame-red sky.

KENNEDY

CHAPTER TEN

Shadows

People said that nothing would grow in Hiroshima for at least seventy-five years after the bomb. This turned out to be untrue. Hiroshima today is shaded by leafy mature trees — willow, cherry, pine. Azaleas bloom along its busy boulevards. Because the center of the city has been preserved as open space and rebuilt as the Peace Park, Hiroshima is, ironically, one of the greenest cities in all of Japan.

In the arrival hall of the Hiroshima train station, I spotted my old friend Shoji right away — though it had been ten years since I'd last seen him. Bearded, black ponytail hanging to his waist, wearing a wrinkled gray Issey Miyake ensemble that looked like a pair of pajamas, he stood out in the crowd. He grinned, grabbing my backpack. "Where's Lloyd?" he asked, puzzled. I explained that he was lying low in a hotel in Tokyo, immobilized by a nasty flu, that I'd only be here in Hiroshima for forty-eight hours.

I met Shoji Kurokami, a Hiroshima native, when he was an art student in Seattle in the early

1980s. In our Seattle days, I'd always admired Shoji's ability to improvise solutions to intractable problems, and his refreshing readiness to embark on spontaneous adventures. Suddenly inspired to attend a Grateful Dead concert in San Francisco? Shoji would jump into his red pickup and, Kerouac-like, drive a thousand miles through the night to get you there.

After finishing art school, Shoji returned to Hiroshima. He married, divorced, and remarried. He and his second wife, Miyuke, have two sons. Divorce is uncommon in Japan, so already Shoji and Miyuke defy the norm. They've built a home in Mukhara-cho, a rural suburb twenty miles north, where Shoji maintains a painting studio and is actively involved in the community.

Currently, Shoji informed me, he was president ("bossman" he called it) of the local PTA. He told me, deadpan, that when another parent complained about a problem at the school, and asked him for his opinion, he advised, "Get rid of education."

What Shoji meant by "education" is the rote authoritarian approach that marked his own elementary and high school experience in Japan. "I believe in curiosity, in encouraging kids to ask questions," he explained. "That's different from 'education,' where they say to student, 'You know nothing. The teacher is only one who knows.' " As a schoolboy in Hiroshima, Shoji refused to cut his hair, wear a school uniform, or join his class in singing *Kimigayo,* the national anthem (a hymn of praise to the emperor).

For Shoji, who is thirty-six, the atom bomb is a fact of life. As a child, he used to wait for the school bus beside a set of concrete steps on the landing of a large downtown bank building. A vague pattern of a human form was etched into the surface. "I always knew there was a human shape there. Citizens can see it every day. So I was pretty shocked when my mother told me it was a 'shadow' and I didn't know what 'shadow' meant."

The intensity of the blast vaporized the human being who sat or stood on those steps on August 6, 1945. The person's body acted as a stencil — briefly masking that spot from the heat and light of the explosion. All that was left of the person was the shadow on the bleached surface. "When I was sixteen," Shoji told me, "they cut the concrete out from the street, lifted it out, and brought it here."

We were standing in front of that same shadow inside the Hiroshima Peace Memorial Museum. Shoji had agreed, somewhat reluctantly, to accompany me. "I come here only once every twenty years," he joked, then looked serious. "My city doesn't have a past," he told me. "Atom bomb wiped that all away."

I described to Shoji the controversy in the States over the Smithsonian exhibit on the dropping of the atom bomb. I told him how, in the words of one Smithsonian official, "the veterans wanted the exhibit to stop when the doors to the bomb bay opened. And that's where the Japanese wanted it to begin."

Shoji considered this, then said thoughtfully, "Who is at fault, who has the guilt, that is not really important issue for me. Peace should be the main issue. The important thing is that as many people see and remember Hiroshima."

He'd heard about the tasteless (and since scrapped) plan for the U.S. Postal Service to issue a stamp showing the mushroom cloud, with the caption, "Hiroshima bomb hastens war's end." Even this didn't faze him. "I can look at stamp in neutral way," he said. "Maybe it helps people to think about Hiroshima. Some people may think bomb was good — and maybe that's OK. But to me, bomb is bomb."

We walked past glass cases containing the devastating relics of the conflagration: a wooden sandal with the imprint of someone's left foot; a carbonized child's lunchbox; the distorted frame of a tricycle that belonged to three-year-old Shimichi Tetsutani, who died in the blast. The legend on the display reads: "Shimichi's father thought his son would be too lonely in the family tomb, so he buried him in the backyard with his best friend, his tricycle." Later, his father dug up the tricycle and donated it to the Peace Museum. I knew Shoji and I were both thinking about Sage, his fearless four-year-old son. That could be Sage's tricycle.

We walked past the life-size diorama of a procession of sufferers against a background of red sky. Skin hung in strips from their flayed arms, which they held out in front of them to ease the pain. We silently observed a photograph of a woman's shoulder, the cross-striped pattern from her kimono permanently imprinted on her skin by the intense heat. Horrifying photos of keloid scars, malformed toenails, women with faces transformed into something resembling bean curd. A piano, a radio, a ten-yen bill. There were sake cups, ivory seals, pipes, teapots, vases — all melted into unrecognizable lumps. A blackened and almost obliterated statue of Daikokutsin had been recovered from a ruined Buddhist temple. Daikokutsin, the caption said, was "the god of good fortune."

This weapon was so insidious, so democratically destructive. The victims' suffering was so grotesque and for many, final.

An uncomfortable thought kept insinuating itself in my mind: part of the story was missing here. I tried to push it away but it bore down with some insistence. There was little introspection here on the larger context of *why* Hiroshima was incinerated, of what else was happening in the world on August 6, 1945. The wording on the Pearl Harbor display was a troubling example: "On December 7, 1941, a bomb was dropped on Pearl Harbor and Japan was hurled into the war." *Was* dropped. *Was* hurled. In this "victims' history," as one scholar called it, "the war appears as a natural catastrophe which 'hap-

166

pened' to Japan, as if without the intervention of human agency."

True, there were some displays downstairs, added as recently as 1994, which showed that Hiroshima was a hub of military activity. But the possible reasons listed in large block type for why the United States dropped the bomb — (1) limiting U.S. casualties, (2) to force Japan to surrender before the Soviet Union could enter the war, and (3) to measure the effectiveness of the bomb — do not mention the responsibility of Japan's own military government's refusal to surrender as a cause.

I had accumulated a collection of books on the subject of Hiroshima and though the debate rages on, what I read had ultimately convinced me that the Japanese military *would not surrender*. Even after the bombing of Nagasaki, on August 9, half the Supreme War Leadership Council was still determined to fight on. War Minister Anami declared to the Cabinet, "I am quite sure that we could inflict great losses on the enemy, and even if we fail in the attempt, our one hundred million people are ready to die with honor." Finally, on August 10, the emperor spoke out and the peace faction on the Cabinet overruled the military zealots. The peace faction considered the atomic bomb to be "a gift from heaven" that allowed them to prevail.

In Luzon, on August 6, 1945, when the war-weary soldiers of the Twenty-fifth Division heard the news of the surrender, they did not

167

know what lay under that mushroom cloud, what lay ahead for the human race and the entire planet as a consequence. At that moment, the bomb meant the end of the war, it meant that they did not have to participate in another bloody campaign. They were going to live, after all.

Paul Fussell, in his essay "Thank God for the Atom Bomb," suggests that "the degree to which Americans register shock and extraordinary shame about the Hiroshima bomb correlates closely with lack of information about the Pacific War." Was this some sort of demented mathematical equation — ten times more knowledge, twenty times less shame? Yet I had to admit that my discomfort about what was missing here was directly related to what I'd learned over the last years about the ghastliness of the Pacific War, and the brutality of Japan's military regime. As I'd talked to Pacific War vets, whenever we came to the subject of the bomb, they would not budge from their implacable belief that its use was absolutely necessary to end the war. The historian Ian Buruma suggests that the attack on Hiroshima might be viewed as "a war crime that actually might have helped to bring the war to a quicker end."

Before we left the museum, I stopped to write in the guest book, waiting first while a woman and her young son made their entries. After they stepped away from the book, I read what the boy, a resident of Hong Kong, had written in a childish scrawl: "I mean, everything here is sad and all, but who started it first? Who attacked other countries first? Who killed first?"

It was not apparent in the museum that, up until the moment the bombs were dropped on Hiroshima and Nagasaki, Japan had been waging a war of aggression.

In a blazing flash, its sins in Korea, Nanking, Burma, and Bataan were dissolved in the greater sins of humankind. In that one instant on August 6, 1945, Japan the aggressor was transformed into Japan the victim. What had gotten lost in that horrific and instantaneous transformation?

We strolled the grounds of Peace Park as a light rain fell. Shoji lit a cigarette as we stood in front of the Peace Cenotaph that contains a box holding the list of the known victims of the bombing. It continues to grow as people die, even now, from radiation sickness. Nearby was a mound of grass under which seventy thousand unidentified bodies lay buried in a mass grave.

"In the years right after 1945, people in Hiroshima really tried to forget about the bombing," Shoji began. "My ex-wife's grandparents — both survivors — didn't tell me anything about the bomb. They just told me a lot about how they recovered. How they planted corn right after the burning." Surprisingly, streetcars were up and running within three days of the blast.

The sight of the functioning streetcars gave hope to the survivors.

"I was raised — almost forced — to believe that America wanted to test a bomb in Japan," Shoji volunteered. Did he believe that? "I do believe that the Americans wanted to use it. They wanted to use it in actual situation. This war was the last chance. The crazy people got a new toy." Did he think the emperor was ready to surrender *before* the bomb was dropped? Shoji paused, "No, I think the emperor really made the decision to surrender because he saw photos of Hiroshima and Nagasaki." Can both of these beliefs be true?

During my visit to Japan, I met Japanese who (unlike Shoji) had lived through the war years. They shocked me when they offered their opinion that the atomic bomb had been necessary to end the war, that the military government would have urged them to mass suicide if the conflagration of Hiroshima hadn't happened.

My veteran friend Baldwin Eckel was one of the first American soldiers to be on Japanese soil after the surrender. He had the opportunity to speak to many high-ranking people associated with the Japanese military industrial complex — officers, government officials, businessmen. To all of them he posed the same question: "What made you willing to surrender?" Every person answered, "Atomic bomb." Baldwin explained to me, "Japan's spiritual fabric was destroyed. It wasn't the Americans who did it. It was the atomic bomb, something supernatural. They could emotionally live with that explanation."

Paul Fussell wrote, "To observe from the viewpoint of the war's victims-to-be that the bomb seemed precisely the right thing to drop is to purchase no immunity from horror." The phrase offers a helpful way to live with two opposing ideas: that the bombing was necessary to bring peace and that the bombing was inexcusable under any circumstances.

Maybe in order to begin to understand Hiroshima, if that is even possible, you have to be willing to live with paradox and contradiction. In Shoji's Zen koan, "Bomb is bomb."

During the war, the Japanese military trained the Special Attack Forces at Etajima, the island across the bay from Hiroshima's Ujina Port. The Imperial Navy Academy was established on Etajima in 1888, and was closed at the end of World War II. It reopened in 1956, as the Japan Maritime Self Defense Force School. I was curious to visit the military museum on Etajima and Shoji agreed to take me there.

The ride on the nearly empty ferry took fifty minutes. The busy harbor, cradled by rolling hills forested with pines, reminded both Shoji and me of Seattle's Puget Sound.

Our tour guide was a genial fellow in a black suit and tie. We were a group of nine, all similarly attired middle-age men except for me and Shoji. From the playing fields in the distance echoed the "hut hut hut!" of the cadets. Clusters of them, all crew cut and lean, jogged past our walking tour.

The guide was in a good mood. One of his remarks provoked laughter from the group. Shoji nudged me with a translation: "He says that American military planned to move into these beautiful buildings at Etajima, that's why they only dropped one bomb on Hiroshima."

Our last stop on the campus was the Educational Museum. We climbed the central marble staircase, which was cloaked in a cascading red carpet. The brochure in English said the museum was intended for students "who come to review the heroic actions of those who have preceded them."

The Nine Heroes of Pearl Harbor were memorialized here, as were the 2,633 Special Attack Forces and kaiten "human torpedo" forces who "died a heroic death." In case after case, as at Yasukuni, the photos and effects of the young pilots were reverentially displayed. Many of them were highly educated young men who were drafted when university deferments were terminated by the government in late 1943.

In 1992, Theodore and Haruko Cook, both historians, published the first oral histories of those few soldiers trained as Special Attack Forces who survived the war. Kozu Noiji was one such survivor:

There are men who returned as many as

four times from missions, but in every case it was because their Kaiten was unable to launch from the host submarine, or no enemy was found. Nobody who was launched from a submarine ever returned, so we don't know their feelings. At that final moment a cold sweat must have broken out. Or maybe they went mad. But there are no witnesses. Nothing could be crueler than that. Nothing.

The word *kaiten* means literally "return to heaven." Theodore Cook describes a kaiten "not so much a ship as an insertion of a human being into a very large torpedo." The "pilot" sat in a canvas chair practically on the deck of the kaiten, a crude periscope directly in front of him, the necessary controls close at hand in the cockpit. The nose assembly was packed with three thousand plus pounds of high explosive; the tail section contained the propulsion unit.

Kozu Noiji received a postcard from a comrade who'd departed on a mission ahead of him: "On it was 'Say hello to Kudo.' That was our code phrase for 'Escape is impossible.' Until that moment we had had no confirmation that the Kaiten was a self-exploding weapon which gave you no chance to escape death."

Kozu had been unable to verify his fears with his fellow cadets, for fear he would disgrace his university. It was a privilege to be chosen for the

Special Attack Forces, a sacrilege to question one's possible fate.

At dusk, we took the ferry back home. The steady hum lulled Shoji to sleep. I stared out the window at the busy tugboats out on the bay.

No American president has apologized for Hiroshima. No Japanese prime minister has directly apologized for Pearl Harbor, or Nanking. Words like *regret* and *remorse* are parsed out by national leaders, and victims understandably find them insufficient. Perhaps my own conflicted feelings inside the Peace Museum were a reflection of the larger ongoing and unresolved debate.

Here's progress, I thought: Before I opened my father's ammo box and found the letters and the flag, I didn't *know* enough to be conflicted. I wished I could have talked to my father about Hiroshima, about how his feelings toward the bombing had changed since that ecstatic day in Luzon in August 1945, when he and his buddies learned the war was over. I felt confident we could have had a good discussion, even a rational discussion.

In *An Ethic for Enemies*, theologian Donald Shriver writes, "In the Peace Museum in Hiroshima, the Japanese mean to show that 'an evil thing happened here. Americans did it.' It may be a half-truth, but it is a truth." Were an American head of state to apologize for Hiroshima, suggested Kenzaburō Ōe, "should he not do so to the children of his country, now and in the future, and the children of the world, and do this because our planet is still haunted by nuclear annihilation?"

The saga of Hiroshima is part of the history (and mythology) of *both* the United States and Japan. As mutual antagonists in a war of relentless carnage, perhaps looking at the whole picture means we have to look at it *together*.

Shriver writes, "The most sober — and hopeful — form of international remembrance is forgiveness, that long, many-sided, seldom-completed process of rehabilitating broken human relationships." Could the Japanese have ended the war sooner? Could the Americans have ended it in any other way? To create the empathy that builds toward forgiveness, shouldn't we ask ourselves — and each other — those questions?

CHAPTER ELEVEN

Amazing Grace

Compared to regions at similar latitude, roughly between that of Casablanca and Barcelona, the west coast of Japan is one of the snowiest places in the world. In winter, cold dry air known as the Siberian High builds up across continental Asia. Part of this air blows eastward from the interior, transforming into northwesterly monsoon winds that gust across the Japan Sea, picking up moisture then dropping it as snow in Japan's central mountain range.

Suibara, a little town of twenty thousand or so souls, is located west of that central mountain range, about thirteen miles inland from the bustling port city of Niigata, in what the Japanese call "the snow country."

We were now, finally, heading toward Suibara. It only took two and a half hours by *shinkansen*, or bullet train, from Tokyo Station to reach Niigata, where we were to spend the night. About an hour into the journey, our sleek train ascended the foothills from the open plain, quilted with the irregular shapes of cultivated fields, and then slipped into a long dark tunnel. I glanced over at Lloyd, who was dozing. I was worried about him. He was still quite ill, his lungs congested, his voice a whisper.

As I looked into the darkness, I began to mull over my encounter the night before with Amy Morita, my only liaison so far with the Shimizu family. We'd met for a curry supper in a Tokyo restaurant. Though it was the first time we'd met in person, it was easy to talk to this frank and warm-hearted young woman. Over chapatis and beer she told me, "I received a call from an official in Suibara a week ago. He wanted to check with me about you, because a few years ago someone from London wanted to return a sword to someone in the town and it turned out they wanted a lot of money for it." I was shocked. Amy continued, "I told them your purpose was strictly personal, and then he asked my advice about what they should do. The Shimizu family is a little panicked, you see. I told them you don't expect anything elaborate. I suggested they think of you like a long-lost friend of their brother."

Then she offered a warning: The Aum guru, Shoko Asahara, had specified April 15 — the day Lloyd and I would be arriving in Suibara — as some kind of doomsday. "No one knows what he has planned. Be very careful," she advised.

Nothing but a sick husband and pending doomsday to worry about, I thought. Suddenly we emerged from the tunnel. A brilliant light flooded our cabin as we headed toward a mountain valley glistening in spring snow.

We spent a restless night in a business hotel in Niigata, a city struck off the atomic bomb target list by the American military a mere three days before they dropped Fat Boy on Hiroshima.

While Lloyd slept, I slipped out to the drab hotel lobby to meet Masako Hayakawa, a local translator who'd volunteered to assist us during our visit to Suibara. Masako was an attractive woman in her fifties, wearing a pleated wool skirt and sensible shoes. She'd studied at the University of Minnesota, majoring in library science, and now lived in nearby Nagaoka, where she worked for the city's international division and taught at local universities. Consummately professional, she exhibited a corresponding kindness that put me at ease.

After briefing me on our itinerary for the next day, Masako used the pay phone in the lobby to call the Shimizu family and confirm we would be arriving the next day by bus. We said our goodnights and I attempted to get some sleep.

The next morning, April 15, I woke up early. The sky had cleared and the day looked promising, no matter what Shoko Asahara had predicted. Lloyd, moving slowly but not complaining, got dressed and ready. At 8:30 A.M. Masako arrived, and we all set off for the bus station.

After hearing Lloyd's hacking cough, Masako detoured our little party to a pharmacy, where she described flu symptoms to the young pharmacist. While she listened to his advice and then purchased some over-the-counter remedies, my eyes took in the familiar shelves of cough syrups, Band-Aids, aspirins. I always feel at home in pharmacies.

I thought about my father, filling prescriptions behind the counter of Edwards Rexall Pharmacy in Culver City. During all those years of listening to stories about other people's pain — all those years of counting out the Valium, the Librium, the Ritalin — did memories of the jungle seep through from time to time?

The bus wound through beautiful countryside — rice paddies and vegetable gardens and old tile-roofed houses. In the distance gleamed the snow-covered Ide mountain range. The bus stopped frequently to pick up passengers — sturdy farmwomen in cotton pants, carrying plastic satchels laden with vegetables. The cherry trees alongside the irrigation canals were in first bloom, and Masako gasped with delight each time we passed a stand of them.

The bus was slow and as the sun warmed my skin, I nodded off. From my half-dream state, a perverse thought bubbled up: Why are you giving up the flag? It belongs to *your* family! Where had *that* come from, I wondered. Before I could answer, Masako cried out with excitement, "We're here! This is our stop!" I was instantly awake. We grabbed our packs, threw our change in the box as Masako instructed, and hopped off the bus.

I was surprised to see two men standing by the side of the road to greet us. They carried signs in Japanese that said, "Welcome to Suibara." The first gentleman was Mr. Asama, from the local Department of Welfare; the other man was Yasue Shimizu, a cousin of Yoshio Shimizu. We filed behind the two men and walked a short distance to the city hall, where the stout and friendly mayor, Mr. Ikarashi, stood waiting next to a shiny black limousine.

More bows. We were introduced to Suezo Shimizu, a courtly man in his sixties with the unruly white hair of an absent-minded professor. He was the husband of Yoshio Shimizu's sister Hiroshi. (He had followed the old custom of taking his wife's surname because her family had lost sons.) Suezo's eyes teared up immediately and so did mine. We bowed deeply. "Ohayo gozaimasu," I said, "Good morning," in handbook Japanese. "O-genki desuka?" ("How are you?") Suezo smiled, speaking rapidly in Japanese, then bowed to Lloyd who extended his hand.

Mr. Mihara, the mayor's eager assistant, opened the door for us. We clambered into the elegant limo with our backpacks. As we drove through the quiet town, we passed people standing on both sides of the street, waving small Japanese and American flags. "Is today some kind of a holiday?" Lloyd asked. Masako translated. The mayor chuckled. "*You* are the occasion," he said. "We are all very touched that you have come from so far away to return the flag."

The mayor informed us that Suibara was so small, it didn't yet have a sister city. The biggest event in tiny Suibara was the yearly arrival of the Siberian swans. The town, I gathered, was like an extended family, so this was really a public, not private, occasion. I was returning the flag to the Shimizu family, but really I was returning the flag to the people of Suibara.

The first thing I noticed as I stepped into the Shimizu house, past the crowd of townspeople, was a simple altar with a framed black-and-white photograph of a young soldier, his face plump and unlined. There he was. Yoshio Shimizu. That's what he looked like.

Lloyd, Masako, and I were ushered to places of honor at the long low table in the center of the room; cups of green tea and sweets shaped like pink lotus awaited us.

Fifty or so people from the neighborhood were crowded into the room. They sat cross-legged on the floor and faced us expectantly, somberly. The mayor sat at the head of the table and he began by introducing the Shimizu family: the three sisters of Yoshio Shimizu — Hiroshi, Hanayo, and Chiyono; Suezo Shimizu; Yasue Shimizu, a first cousin; and the son of Yoshio Shimizu's older brother, Yoshinobu Shimizu, in whose house we were all gathered. Yoshinobu was a robust young man with glossy black hair that stood straight up from his head. His two-year-old daughter sat comfortably in her daddy's lap, observing the event with great solemnity.

Out of the corner of my eye, I gratefully noted that Lloyd, despite his flu haze, had stepped into his role as official photographer. He moved around the room with fluid grace, snapping shots from various positions.

There was an air of electric emotion in the room. When I raised my cup of tea to take a sip, I noticed that my hand was shaking. Masako nodded at me; it was the moment to hand over the flag.

On the bus ride to Suibara, I was gripped by an irrational fear that the box in my backpack was empty, that somehow I had forgotten to take the flag or had left it in the hotel in Tokyo, or on the train to Niigata. I was suddenly terrified that I'd unzip the backpack and there would be nothing inside. I couldn't bring myself to check at the time.

Now I reached into the backpack, felt the contours of the box, and pulled it out. I placed it on the table in front of Hiroshi, whose birth order in the family placed her closest to Yoshio among the surviving siblings.

Hiroshi opened the box with her gnarled hands and drew out the flag. A collective gasp. Then crying. Then applause. "Show it to everyone!" exclaimed the mayor. Hiroshi spread the square of silk on the table. There it was — an incontrovertible fact. "I realize seeing this flag again may make you feel sad," I said softly, "but I hope it will help you honor the memory of your brother." Hanayo dabbed her wet eyes with a handkerchief.

The mayor then presented me with four large wrapped boxes, explaining that they were a gift of appreciation from the town. I started to open the first when the room began to clatter and shudder. No one budged. I sat frozen to the tatami mat.

After what felt like a full minute, the room ceased to vibrate. Everybody cautiously smiled at one other. There. We'd been through something together. Instead of ratcheting up the emotional tenor, the earthquake lent the room a new calm. We all sat quietly without speaking for several moments, a mutual acknowledgment of forces beyond our control. When it was clear that the temblor was over, smiles broke out on many faces.

I opened the boxes. Inside the first box were three traditional "Dharma" dolls, made by a hundred-year-old Suibara craftsman. They were shaped like the conical hats Suibara children traditionally wear to ward off snow. In the second box, a dozen beautiful pastries shaped like swan eggs. In the third was a brooch in the shape of a swan. Inside the fourth box was a framed photograph of swans in flight.

Three of the men in the room stood and introduced themselves. Masako translated: "We were all the same age as Yoshio. We lived in the same neighborhood. Yuko was the oldest and Yoshio was the youngest of the four. But Yoshio was the tallest and was one of the nice-looking young men and he was most popular with the girls! He was a very gentle and kind person." Yoshio was eighteen when he left to fight in the Japanese Imperial Army. He was twenty-one when his family received word he had died. His sister told me, "We didn't know if he was killed on a ship or on the land. It was quite difficult to learn how he died, how he was killed. At that time it was difficult to get any kind of information."

Masako had warned me the family would probably want to know how my father got the flag. One of the elderly men posed the question. "I can't say for sure. I wish that I could," I said. I explained that my father regretted sending the flag home. That he informed my mother of his regret over and over again. That he probably gathered it up from items left behind in a cave by retreating Japanese soldiers. No one pressed the issue, yet the question hovered in the air. Perhaps, I thought in hindsight, I was fortunate not to possess a conclusive answer.

Masako translated one man's thoughtful offering: "You must understand. For those of us who were in the war, when we see the flag before us, it makes our hearts ache." I looked at these aging men. I wondered what horrors they had endured or possibly, in the name of the emperor, might have inflicted on Chinese or Filipino civilians, or British POWs. I wondered what conflicts from their war service continued to plague their minds and dreams. One man had served in Manchuria, another in Mindanao. They possessed memories they had probably never shared with their wives or children. I couldn't assure these men that my father had not been the one who killed their friend Yoshio Shimizu, that he hadn't taken that flag from his dead body. The "tragic irony of war," as Amy Morita had called it, resonated throughout the room.

The mayor asked Lloyd to say a few words. Bleary with fever, assailed by emotions, and constricted by the formality of the situation, he managed a few sentences until his gracious hosts let him off the hook.

After the speeches, the women working behind the scenes brought out an enormous banquet: platters of colorful sushi, tempura, crab's legs, and red-bean rice, made specially for auspicious occasions. The men chain-smoked American cigarettes. Bottles of beer and carafes of sake appeared. The tone in the room changed. There was laughter, joking. The men came over to slap Lloyd on the back. Our glasses were always full.

The flag was fondled, caressed, examined. "Do you remember where you signed? Look here!" Several people found their names on the flag, where they signed fifty years ago — offering the young soldier good luck as he departed for a foreign land. This kind of flag is called *yosegaki*, which means a collection. A collection of names.

The Shimizu family had embraced the advice that Amy Morita had given them — to think of us as the long-lost friends of the missing soldier. Heady from my never-empty glass of sake and the thrill of this gathering, I felt as though we were.

I remembered that it was the first night of the Jewish holiday of Passover and we were the honored guests at the banquet, just as I had imagined Yoshio Shimizu as the honored guest at my father's seder in the middle of a war.

The words we repeat each year at Passover as part of the service took on new meaning: "Since you were once a stranger in the land of Egypt, thou shalt love the stranger as thyself."

By late afternoon, the gathering finally started to break up. The house emptied as everyone left and assembled in the driveway for a group photo. Two lawn chairs were brought out for Lloyd and me. Yoshio's three sisters knelt down on the ground to my right. The elder men, including Suezo and the mayor, squatted to Lloyd's left. Yoshinobu, his two-year-old perched on his shoulder, stood directly behind us. In front of him, between Lloyd and me, his wife cradled their youngest. Four of Yoshio's old friends held the flag, each one gripping a corner of the silk square. Masako took the left flank. Click. The moment was recorded: We now shared a common history.

★ ★ ★

The Shimizus and the mayor were eager to take us to Lake Hyoko, Suibara's premier tourist destination, and introduce us to the Swan Uncle, one of the town's most respected citizens. Masako filled me in on the story of Suibara and its swans.

Until the late nineteenth century, Suibara had been the seasonal home to five-foot-tall whooper swans that arrived each fall from Siberia to escape the rigors of the northern winter. They wintered on Suibara's reservoir lake, limned with pine trees that created a natural windscreen. The townspeople considered the birds "honored guests"; hunting them was strictly forbidden. Each spring, the swans migrated back to their nesting grounds in the Siberian tundra.

After Japan opened to trade with the West, firearms, originally introduced by Portuguese sailors in the fifteenth century, were distributed widely throughout the country. The villagers of Suibara began to hunt the once-protected birds. Tokyo shops paid high prices for swan meat, which was considered a delicacy. About the same time, noisy factories sprouted up on land that had been rice paddies, their waste emptying into lakes and wetlands in Niigata Prefecture. The combination of hunting pressure and habitat loss ultimately proved too much for the whooper swans. By the early 1900s, they disappeared altogether from Suibara.

In 1950, inexplicably, after an absence of four

decades, eight whooper swans returned to Hyoko Lake from their summer nesting grounds in the Siberian tundra. The villagers were amazed to see the spectacular birds adrift on their lake. They crowded along the shoreline, shouting. Some ran for their guns. The shy birds, alarmed, took off. If it hadn't been for one very determined man, a farmer named Jusaburo Yoshikawa, they might never have returned.

Yoshikawa dedicated his life to persuading his neighbors to leave the swans in peace, and persuading the whoopers to stay in Suibara. He patiently patrolled the lake day and night, exhorting villagers to avoid frightening the swans. When the lake froze over, he hacked through the ice with an ax, wading out in hip-high boots to clear away the shards so the swans could forage for oat grass on the lake bottom.

Yoshikawa's single-minded efforts originally earned him the title of Swan Fool from his fellow villagers. His wife, whom he persuaded to make daily requests of local grocers for discarded greens for the swans, was called the Swan Widow. But he eventually managed to get Lake Hyoko declared a protected zone, officially the "Winter Habitat of Wild Swans at Suibara"; and that same year, 1954, he received the title of Swan Father. His son, Shigeo, who carried on his father's tradition of caring for the swans, is known as the Swan Uncle.

The magnificent whoopers are now little Suibara's main claim to fame. Their return was

Suibara's good omen and then its postwar recovery miracle, bringing thousands of Japanese tourists to the town each winter. The townspeople are both grateful and protective. Schoolchildren in Suibara form swan patrols to assist with feedings, and to insure that the birds are not harassed.

We sat in the observation room at the lake's feeding station with Shigeo Yoshikawa, the bespectacled Swan Uncle. Nori machi, a green tea that tastes like chicken soup, was served. Exhausted from the emotion of the afternoon, no one ventured small talk. We all stared out the windows, looking one way toward a field of purple irises, the other way toward the lake and those few swans still in spring residence; their black-beaked beauty was startling against the pale reeds. "Louise-san must come back in swan season," Shigeo announced, with a voice of quiet insistence. The Shimizus all nodded enthusiastically. The idea appealed to me, unlikely as it seemed. Then it was time to go.

The Shimizu family insisted on driving Lloyd, Masako, and me the forty minutes to the Niigata train station. Once we'd located the right track and the right shinkansen train and seated ourselves inside on the correct seats, the family assembled outside the window, the colors of their sweaters and jackets making a somber study in mauves, blues, and gray.

They did not wave, but stayed in their places as if a portrait photographer were taking a long exposure. The women were in the front, the men behind them. Hiroshi, Hanayo, and Chiyono — the three sisters of Yoshio Shimizu — stood elbow to elbow, their hands clasped together and their pocketbooks over their forearms. Behind them: Hiroshi's husband, Suezo; cousin Yasue, the farmer; and beside him, the new patriarch, young Yoshinobu, Yoshio's nephew.

I kept my eyes on the assembled family as the train pulled out of the station. I was relieved that Yoshio's flag was now in their possession — home where it belonged.

PART III

The Philippines

CHAPTER TWELVE

The American Cemetery

A few days later, on the plane to Manila, I kept thinking about the Shimizu family, standing outside our train compartment window.

I tried to sleep. Lloyd and I were both exhausted. Lloyd was barely recovered from the flu. I wasn't sure we had the stamina for Manila in the hot season, and for the journey to the site in the mountains of northern Luzon, where my father assumed guardianship of the flag.

Reading the warnings in *The Lonely Planet* guidebook did not do much to spark our enthusiasm for travel: "Beware of pickpockets, thieving cabbies, strangers who offer drugged sweets, or drunks."

I'd already inherited an antipathy to the Philippines, reinforced by my father's letters.

10 September 1945
When I get home, I never want to be reminded of the Philippines. Everything on this island will always bring back sad memories and remind me of six long months of

hell — living in fear — seeing such horrible sights day in and especially the nights of being awake and always on guard wondering and waiting.

That same September, in Luzon before his division left for Japan, he made a sobering trip to the cemetery in the barrio of Santa Barbara. He brought his camera: "Many of the pictures I took were of the boys that I knew and some of the entire cemetery as a whole."

He went to visit the still-fresh graves of friends like Sam Wengrow, "the Jewish lad from Florida." Sam had been killed by a sniper on May 29, 1945, after the Battle of Balete Pass was officially over.

17 September 1945

Yesterday I went on that trip to the cemetery in Santa Barbara. I'm very glad that I went. It will always remain with me. The thousands of symmetric white crosses and Stars of David sprinkled in between. It was very impressive and very sobering.

Richard's and Sam's graves didn't even have their names or dog tags on their crosses — we just figured it out by the sequence of numbers and then I went to the office and made sure that they'll change Sam's cross to a Star of David. Not that it matters much to Sam now — but since his faith was Hebrew — I thought it would be more fitting.

194

Some of the graves were just marked unknown — quite a few of them — and as I've said before there really are many Stars. Most of the boys that came out of my outfit didn't know what the Stars were for. So I explained that to them.

After the war, the American Military Cemetery in Manila was designated as the permanent resting place for Americans who died in the Philippine campaign, and soldiers buried at several sites around the Philippines, including the cemetery in Santa Barbara, were reinterred here.

Our accommodations were reserved at the Midland Plaza Hotel in downtown Manila, an unlovely modern behemoth, thirty floors of gray concrete with a shiny marble lobby, uniformed elevator men, and its own coffee shop.

The hotel was a leftover from Marcos's heyday, and tourist business must have been slow. No other guests in that vast building ever revealed themselves to us during our entire stay. No one else appeared in the coffee shop, no one else but us cashed traveler's checks at the front desk. The management must have rented out the rooms to long-term guests. We smelled curries simmering and heard families arguing behind closed doors in the long carpeted corridor.

The security guards chatting in the lobby were armed with semiautomatics. There had been a recent spate of bank robberies in Manila, which were thought to be linked to the guerrilla movement on the southern islands. The hotel porter, a sweet young man named Louis, insisted on walking us the half block to the 7-Eleven, where we bought midnight snacks before turning in. The security guard at the 7-Eleven was fondling a semiautomatic as well.

Our room was really a suite, with two huge rooms and a balcony overlooking Manila Harbor. In Japan, all of the hotel rooms we stayed in would have fit inside this one. And it was cheap, too, by American standards. In fact, after Japan, where buying a cantaloupe was like trading in stocks and bonds, Filipino currency was like Monopoly money. Our first night we both slept fitfully, each waking up several times to the sound of the rasping air conditioner.

In the morning, we had coffee and toast in the Midland Hotel coffee shop, which doubled in the evening hours as a nightclub. Its most distinguishing feature was the painted mural of American movie stars — Marilyn on the ski slope, James Dean lounging, Fred and Ginger (who sported a chapeau resembling a plate of scrambled eggs) dancing the night away.

When we stepped outside the air-conditioned hotel, the force of mid-morning heat nearly knocked us over. We made our way toward the bay, past tiny foodstands selling snacks I wouldn't dare eat: pickled pigs' feet and jars of large eggs glistened in the hot sun. Whenever we stopped, a jeepney — one of Manila's garishly decorated local vans — slammed on its brakes beside us, the driver shouting out, "Want a ride?" As tourists, we stood out.

Trying to get across a boulevard took nerve. None of the stoplights were working, and the flow of jeepneys and taxis and buses was constant and thick. So was the air, wretched with exhaust.

A nine-year-old in rags, his scrawny brother on his back, darted among the cars with his hand outstretched. Lloyd pressed a twenty-peso bill into it, and the boy retreated to the shade of the crosswalk. Maybe it bought him a few minutes' rest. Another boy working the intersection dragged his withered leg. A third beggar had no legs at all, just a crumbled stump of a torso. Acupuncture needles adorned his ears. Manila was a carnival of pain.

On the bay side of the boulevard, families rested under the scraggly coconut palms. People were swimming in the murky water. We passed several horse-drawn carriages, intended for tourists. The ponies looked half-dead. They shifted their weight from front foot to back, their shaggy heads held low. The driver ran after us: Did we want a ride? No? Maybe later? No? How long were we staying? At what hotel?

We wandered into the old Malate cathedral, a colonial leftover, just before Sunday morning mass. Portable fans purred away, stirring the air around the parishioners. Doleful statues of suffering Christ watched over them. I was relieved to sit down and rest on a hard wooden pew in the peaceful sanctuary. Sparrows flitted through the interior, perching on the unlit chandeliers. A plastic bag floated down the aisle, propelled by the breeze. I watched the neatly dressed families: young mothers and fathers with four, five young children each, each child's hair combed and braided. The priest announced in an Irish accent, "Christ is alive and Christ loves us." A neon sign by the altar — "Jesus Loves You" — blinked on and off.

In Japan, after Lloyd became ill, I had taken the lead, making sure he got sleep, procuring hot drinks, coercing him into seeing the sights, making sure we got to our trains and got off them at the right time. Here, light-headed from the heat, I was the more fragile one. Lloyd, beginning to feel normal, took over the practical details: He navigated, checked timetables, consulted maps, paid taxi drivers. I sat in the pew and concentrated my thoughts on the story Masako's husband told me.

After leaving Suibara, Lloyd and I had stayed overnight at their home. On the train ride there, Masako had mentioned that her husband, Norio, an engineering professor, had an unusual war story. "But he never talks about it," she said.

When we got to her house, Norio met us at the door. He had a boyish grin and wore at-home clothes — jeans and a comfy sweater. After a spaghetti dinner, we settled into conversation. Norio was listening intently to the story of the flag and our visit with the Shimizu family. At one point he excused himself and returned with a tattered photo album. He set it down on the coffee table, then lifted out a photo of a young couple and their infant son.

The couple was strikingly handsome. The husband had a crisp part in his hair. He wore an elegant suit. His delicate wife wore a traditional silk kimono. Norio stared at it before handing it to me. "These are my parents," he explained.

The photo was taken in 1939, three years after his parents had been posted to Manchuria. His young father was an official of the Manchuko (puppet) government, established by the Japanese to rule over China. Settling in Manchuria was considered both a patriotic duty and an adventurous opportunity.

Norio was born there. He was six when, just before the war officially ended, the Russians invaded. His father was arrested, one of an estimated 1.3 million Japanese who fell into Soviet hands. He was taken to a Siberian concentration camp and never heard from again, along with three hundred thousand Japanese never accounted for after the war. His mother died in China a year later, during a cholera epidemic. A great-uncle brought Norio back to Japan along with his own children, and another uncle raised him.

Over the past decade, academic conferences and engineering consultations had taken Norio to China on several occasions. On a recent trip, he'd decided to find the apartment where, as he put it, "I lost my mother." He only had a vague memory of the place where the sick woman bade her son farewell, but with the help of Chinese friends who knew the town, he somehow found it. "Were you flooded with memories?" I asked him. He sighed. "That only happens in novels."

His success in finding his mother's last resting place released something in him. He then decided to go to Siberia to find his father's grave. He'd always assumed his father had died in the camp. "I really didn't want to go," he told me, "but I felt I had to."

In order to find the place where the camp had once been located, Norio first took a train across the Siberian taiga, then a boat ride along the Amur River, then a bus ride along a wooded area to a small village. From that village a small, hired bus took him to a forested hill a few miles away, where he waited for a rendezvous with a logging truck. When it showed up, he clambered aboard and they rolled through the rutted and muddy woods to a murky, deserted lake surrounded by straggly conifers. It was so quiet. This place was generally acknowledged as the site where the prison camp had been in the forties and fifties. The rig pulled off the muddy road and the trucker turned off the motor, lit a cigarette, and grunted, "Over there." Norio climbed out of the truck and walked into the thicket of pines. There, the son finally saw with his own eyes what passed for his father's grave: three foot by three foot pits here and there where, fifty years ago, according to the local villagers, the bodies of ninety Japanese prisoners had been unceremoniously dumped.

There was a long awkward silence after Norio had told me this, the kind that comes after someone has revealed something intimate to a stranger. Norio stared at the photo of his parents. I could think of no way to call him back out of his painful reverie. We simply sat there, listening to the clock ticking until we said our goodnights and then went to bed.

In the middle of the night, I woke up and slid open the wooden door to the darkened living room. There on the coffee table was the tattered photo of the young couple and their beautiful infant son. I sat down, picked up the photo and studied it. I wondered if Norio, while standing in that muddy spot in the Siberian woods, had conducted some kind of religious service. Did he pray or did he curse? Or was it enough that he was simply *there?*

The mass at Malate was over; the warm air was sweet with the smell of incense. The parishioners filed outside and the pink-cheeked priest smiled at each of them as they left. Outside the cathedral, Lloyd hailed a cab and three came screeching to a halt. "For American Cemetery. Fort Bonifacio," he said.

The driver immediately turned up the volume on his radio and began singing along with the

American pop songs about lost love. At breakneck speed, he drove us through the crowded barrios. One slum was adorned with a huge billboard showing the Pope kissing a baby and admonishing everyone to "Honor Life." Hollow-eyed children hawked strings of white flower blossoms to the honking drivers stalled at intersections. We drove past a statue of Senator Benigno (Ninoy) Aquino, Filipino patriot and opposition leader, who was shown with a dove on his shoulder and his hand extended in a handshake — frozen in the moment he returned to Manila from exile in the United States on August 21, 1983. On that clear Sunday afternoon with thousands of supporters waiting, he was gunned down on the airport tarmac. The dictator Marcos was universally assumed to be the one who ordered his rival's assassination.

We passed huge department stores and a nearly empty downtown. We skirted a neighborhood of garish mansions behind electric gates. The cab carried us into Fort Bonifacio, the former military camp (where Ninoy Aquino had spent eight years in solitary confinement) that was decommissioned and is now a golf course and country club, and finally through the gates of the American Cemetery.

It was a lush, green world far from the bleak density of Manila's slums. Here, 17,206 Americans — the largest number of our World War II military dead — rested on 152 acres landscaped with massive carob trees, flame trees, and coral

trees from India. Mahogany trees from Mada-
gascar shaded lawns as immaculate as putting
greens. Unlike the rest of Manila, the cemetery
had its own water purification system; mourners
are provided with potable water.

Lloyd and I walked across the vast arrangement of graves. There was an immaculate order
to the place, the headstones arranged in con-
centric circular rows. The guidebook said that
of the total, "13,434 headstones marked the
graves of single identified remains; 6 marked
the graves of 28 identified remains that could
not be separated individually; 3,644 marked
the graves of single unidentified remains (Un-
knowns) and 16 marked the graves of 100 unidentified remains that could not be separated
individually." Remains. All that was left of humans who were sons and brothers, fathers and
grandfathers, uncles and nephews, friends and
neighbors. Every hour the carillon tolled, followed by two military songs — familiar but un-
identifiable.

In my knapsack were several photographs my
father had taken on that September day in 1945,
when he visited the cemetery in the barrio of
Santa Barbara, where his friends had been hast-
ily buried. Before we'd left L.A., Lloyd had
printed and enlarged some of the negatives so
that we could read the names on the headstones.
In the photos, the graves looked achingly raw.

We walked through the acres of grave markers,
examining as many with Stars of David on them

as we could, hoping against hope to find the grave of one of the buddies my father had mentioned in his letters or whose name was in one of the headstone photos.

We passed headstones with Stars of David that belonged to Milton Tepper; Harry Fineman; Sol Margolis; Max Biederman, but no one whose name my father had mentioned. We walked by many blank markers that said, simply, "Here Rests in Honored Glory / A Comrade in Arms / Known but to God."

At the visitors' center, a groundskeeper noticed us and asked if he could help. He pulled out a huge three-ring binder and asked us what names we were hoping to find. He ran his callused finger down a long list and stopped in the W section. "I will take you there," he offered. He motioned to a motorcycle with a sidecar. We motored through the cemetery, agog at the sheer size of the place. There were headstones as far as the eye could see.

Mr. Rocaberte stopped the motorcycle and pointed. Lloyd and I stepped out of the sidecar and walked toward the Jewish star with "Sam Wengrow" carved on it. I was surprised at the amount of emotion this grave brought up in me. I'd never known Sam Wengrow.

When he returned home from the war, my father wanted to "bury" his memories. But when he stood in front Sam's grave, as an expression of respect, he vowed to keep that visit "always with him." His desires were irreconcilable: He wanted to never forget and he needed to never remember.

I'd asked my war veteran mentor Baldwin Eckel why he never talked about his war experiences to his family, or to anyone:

You talk to any veteran who has been in real combat, and see how much he talks about it. It's so painful, so much anguish. It's not the enemy dying. That's nothing. It's your buddies. And it leaves scars that you just can't talk about.

In one skirmish I was next to a lieutenant, who was killed. He was a good buddy of mine. We were real close. That was such a painful experience for me. After that, I never called anybody by their name. It was always by their rank. Colonel. Captain. General. Soldier. Private. Sergeant. That was my way of protecting myself. *I know nobody's name.*

Had my father been able to share his grief for Sam? Had he *ever* been able to weep? His closest buddies in combat were like family. He had lost family before. The pain of his childhood loss reverberated with each friend's death in combat.

Mr. Rocaberte stepped back by his motorcycle to wait while I pulled out a prayer book and murmured the kaddish. Lloyd said out loud, "Sam, I don't think anyone has visited you in a long time, but we're here now." I wondered if Sam

Wengrow's family had been to Manila. I thought of my aunt Ruth's grave somewhere in Queens, and vowed to make a visit there. Lloyd bent down and ran his hands over the marble headstone, "See ya later, Sam," he whispered.

The gently sloping lawns led to a memorial hall at the top of the hill. In each room of the hall was a mural map of the various campaigns of the Pacific War, and a list of those who died in each. In the room that included the map of the Luzon Campaign, I examined the guest book. I read the following entries, made that same day:

"We are the world."
"No more wars."
"My dad would be proud."
"Very impressive."
"This place makes me feel sad."
"Make love not war."

A Japanese family, two young parents and their sons, were visiting the memorial hall at the same time. I wondered if they felt as strange here as I'd felt at the Peace Memorial in Hiroshima.

I opened the guest book to a blank page and wrote, "We are here to honor my father and his comrades from the 25th Infantry 'Tropic Lightning' Division, 27th Regiment, who fought in the battle for Balete Pass."

CHAPTER THIRTEEN

Journey to Balete Pass

Balete Pass is the lowest point (3,000 feet) in the long, jumbled complex of ridges that make up the Caraballo Mountains in northern Luzon. The highest point of this rugged range, Mount Imugan, crests at 5,580 feet. It is through narrow (75 feet across) Balete Pass that Luzon's main artery, National Highway 5, passes over the Caraballos. "Balete Pass is located at the northern exits of the most tortuous terrain Route 5 traverses on its way north," states the *War in the Pacific* volume of the official U.S. Army chronicle on World War II. The pass is the gateway to the fertile rice fields of the Cagayan Valley, and during the war, as one salty vet put it, "it was the dividing line, real estatewise."

In 1944, it was General MacArthur's unalterable belief that the Allies should secure Luzon before moving any closer to an invasion of Japan. This belief put General MacArthur at odds with the Navy High Command, who advocated bypassing Luzon for an assault on Formosa.

MacArthur had political as well as military

motives. In 1942, American troops had suffered a historic defeat in the Philippines at the hands of the Japanese. MacArthur's famous vow — "I shall return," made on March 11, 1942, when he left Corregidor and evacuated to Australia on FDR's orders — was viewed by Filipinos, under Japanese occupation, with quasi-mystical status. MacArthur considered the reoccupation of the entire Philippine archipelago a "national obligation."

MacArthur's argument eventually won the debate among the Joint Chiefs of Staff. U.S. forces would bypass Formosa and recapture the Philippines in a consecutive series of advances, just as MacArthur had been planning since March 1942.

As part of MacArthur's overall strategy, Lieutenant General Walter Krueger, the United States Sixth Army commander on Luzon, ordered the Twenty-fifth "Tropic Lightning" Division to launch the drive to secure Balete Pass from the Japanese. From General Krueger to General Mullins, Commander of the Twenty-fifth Division; from General Mullins to General Dalton, Assistant Commander of the Twenty-fifth; from General Dalton to innumerable colonels, majors, captains, and so on down the chain of command — MacArthur's strategy ultimately brought infantrymen like my father and his comrades, as well as vets like Sylvan Katz and Peter Lomenzo and Baldwin Eckel, to northern Luzon to put their lives on the line to stop the Japanese.

The objective was to cut off General Yamashita's forces from rice fields in the Cagayan Valley. Since rice was the mainstay of the Imperial Army during the war, the objective was clear: Deprive the enemy of access to the "rice bowl," and the campaign would be won.

Known as the Tiger of Malaya for capturing Singapore, General Tomoyuki Yamashita was both brilliant and realistic as a military strategist. He did not anticipate winning any major battles, or even driving the Americans away. By ceding Manila and the Central Plains and withdrawing the bulk of his Fourteenth Area Army, a force of more than 150,000 men, into the nearly impregnable Caraballos, he aimed to make the Americans pay dearly for their victory. Yamashita was determined to delay the conquest of Luzon as long as possible in order to pin down as many U.S. divisions as he could, to slow the Allied advance toward Japan. The longer he could keep the American infantry and its air support tied up in combat, the longer the home islands would have to prepare for the inevitable Allied invasion. (Ironically, this strategy also gave the Americans more time to ready the atomic bomb.)

The Luzon Campaign was the largest of the Pacific War, employing the use of more United States Army ground combat and service forces than those used in operations in North Africa, Italy, or southern France. The victory at Balete Pass severed Yamashita's troops from their food supplies, the fatal blow to Japanese resistance on Luzon. The battle itself set a record for consecutive days of combat in the Pacific War. Radio reports in 1945 termed it a "second Cassino," in reference to the brutal, decisive land battle in Italy that claimed so many Allied lives in the European theater. Yet, the battle for Balete Pass, vital to victory in the Philippines, is seldom mentioned in most histories of the Pacific War.

In a 1998 issue of *World War Two* magazine, one military historian wrote of the Twenty-fifth Division and Balete Pass, "Its accomplishment is obscured by MacArthur's pronouncement that the Philippines had been secured as early as March. The Twenty-fifth had a victory in a war that trumpeted victories, and yet its dead and wounded remain largely forgotten."

We left Manila on a small, crowded plane and flew north to Baguio, in the mountains of northern Luzon. From Baguio, we figured, we could drive to Balete Pass in a day.

Situated at a mile-high elevation among fragrant pine forests, Baguio was designated the summer capital of the Philippine Archipelago by the American colonial government in 1903. It is at least twenty degrees cooler than Manila, which is why it is always crowded with urbanites who have either moved here or can afford to make it their summer destination.

On December 8, 1941, schoolchildren in Baguio lining up for their morning assembly were surprised to hear the sound of planes over-head, and even more shocked when Japanese bombs rained from the sky. Directly in the path of the Japanese invasion of Luzon, Baguio was the Imperial Army's next target after Pearl Harbor, and Japanese troops quickly overran the ruined town. They converted Camp John Hay, the once-verdant park containing American officers' residences, into their garrison and designated part of it as an internment camp for about five hundred Allied citizens — including Americans, Canadians, British nationals, and Australians.

After the Japanese attack in 1941, many Baguio residents escaped into the mountains to join bands of Filipino guerrilla forces, who were later instrumental in helping the Americans liberate the island.

During the short plane ride, we tried to locate Balete Pass on our map. It wasn't there. We pinpointed the area where it should have been. No such place-name existed. The plane began its descent. "Well," Lloyd conceded, "it's not like going to Gettysburg."

At the little Baguio airport, cabbies vied for our fare. A pockmarked driver named Joey, the most assertive, quickly loaded our backpacks into his trunk, and in minutes we were lurching toward Baguio in his fender-bent '72 Toyota.

Joey had big plans for our visit. He would be our personal chauffeur and tour guide deluxe. He would take us to special nightclubs and private cockfights. On a lark, Lloyd asked, "Can you take us to Balete Pass?" Joey looked puzzled for a moment, then brightened up. "Ah! You mean Dalton Pass!" he exclaimed, pulling deeply on a Marlboro. "They changed the name after that general got killed."

Brigadier General James L. "Rusty" Dalton II, the popular Assistant Division Commander of the Twenty-fifth Infantry, was on a reconnaissance mission at Balete Pass on May 16, 1945, when he was felled by a sniper's bullet to the back of the head.

Just thirty-six years old when he was killed, Dalton had been one of the army's youngest generals. In a published interview, General Stanley "Swede" Larsen, Dalton's fellow officer in the Twenty-fifth, remembered him as "a hell of a nice fellow." After Dalton's untimely death, his soldiers, still in their combat garb, honored their general with a Requiem Mass and then buried him in an emotional ceremony at the army cemetery near Santa Barbara, Luzon.

Dalton's death stunned the entire division, and, according to Peter Lomenzo, it inspired the bone-weary men of the Twenty-fifth to fight even harder. For even with Balete Pass finally secured, the division faced more combat. Not until the last day of June did the Twenty-fifth Division complete their final phase of the Luzon Campaign, "eliminating" (less euphemistic than "mopping up") the last concentrations of "fanatically resisting" Japanese.

Dalton Pass was not on Joey's list of hot spots around Baguio, but he was excited at the idea that we might hire him to take us there. At least he tried to convince Lloyd that he was the man for the job. "It's an all-day trip," he said. "But I'll take you to see faith healers, too . . . for a little extra."

Neither Joey's dervishlike driving style nor the absence of shocks in his cab inspired confidence as we careened up the twisting roads to Baguio. The cab shuddered to a halt in front of our hotel, a rustic inn on a side street.

Joey lingered in the lobby until we started up the staircase toward our room, carrying our bags. "I come back in morning," Joey told Lloyd confidently. "I take you to Dalton Pass. One hundred dollars for whole day. I am yours."

I gave my husband a not-so-subtle elbow in the ribs. It was true — we did want a driver. Three days in Manila had convinced both of us that we were not cut out to drive in the Philippines. We could barely make it across the street. But I did not want Joey to be "ours" for the whole day; I did not want us to be "his." Joey was insistent. "I'll be here early in morning," he yelled, rattling off in a cloud of noxious fumes.

The hotel staff recommended someone named Arnel Fetilano as a potential driver and guide. Arnel operated a fledgling travel service out of Baguio. He came over, and in the Chinese restaurant adjacent to the hotel, we spread our maps out on the table. Arnel assured us that we'd made the right choice in deciding not to do the driving ourselves. Large portions of the road to Balete (Dalton) Pass were damaged by earthquake, others by a recent typhoon.

I told Arnel, a slender young man with a studious air, that we wanted to go to Dalton Pass because my father had fought a battle there. He nodded. "My mother lived in the forest near Dalton Pass during the war," he told me. "My grandfather was with the guerrilleros." We made a plan: Arnel would pick up his friend's Dodge Caravan and be at our hotel the next morning.

That night, anxious about the next day's expedition, we tried to sleep as a light summer rain tapped on our windows.

Around nine A.M., Arnel pulled up in a large, boxy van and we set off. What would take us nearly fourteen hours to traverse round-trip (about 140 miles) took the Twenty-fifth Infantry Division, beginning in January 1945, 165 days, one way.

We drove northward through a deep, sharp-sided river valley. On the side of the road, old women sold bananas, peanuts, and mangos. Brightly painted jeepneys, packed to capacity, clattered by in the opposite direction. We passed a boy herding piglets, groups of children playing, women sitting in chairs under stilted, thatched huts grooming one another's hair.

We emerged from the valley onto a flat plain, with fields stretching far off into the distance on both sides. The landscape of the Luzon plain had changed little from my father's descriptions of it half a century ago. The solid shapes of carabao, the ubiquitous ox of the Philippines, dotted the dry rice paddies. "A carabao is as strong as an elephant," Arnel informed us proudly. Inside the air-conditioned van, we rode in cool comfort. Outside, the temperature rose steadily.

On the night of January 18, 1945, on the same open plain, my father lay awake in the foxhole he shared with Morrie Franklin, another GI, trying not to move at all.

> Due to the strain we've been under, some of the boys sometimes get nightmares at night. Luckily I haven't had any, but Morrie Franklin, the lad I usually sleep with these nights, said that I do mumble in my sleep. One night he thought I had asked him a question and when he looked at me, he realized I was asleep.

A jungle night bird rapping on a tree trunk put my father's nerves on edge. It could be the enemy knocking out a code on bamboo sticks. He startled at the sound of leaves rustling, his finger on the trigger of his rifle. What felt like an hour passed. He glanced again at his watch. Just a few minutes had elapsed.

215

My father wished he could write by the light of the moon, but he knew that "no one is safe if he moves about." He waited until morning to write.

27 January 1945

While I'm writing a young mother is feeding her baby at the breast very uninhibited and a young lad about five is looking for lice in her hair — one of their favorite pastimes is delousing each other. Another of their favorite activities is watching us while we take a bath. It seems as though no one is around when we start but before long we can see faces staring at us from all over. Of course we're getting used to it.

Today four of us came across a native home and sent a little boy up a coconut tree. Gosh it was tall. Up he went like a monkey and we had juice and the shell. They really treat you friendly. And then they bring out bananas and offer apologies when we ask for eggs and they don't have any to give us.

When we're on the move, they stand along the road and yell "Victoree" and something that sounds like "Ah bouhai." That means Hurrah.

Not until the final paragraph does he confess his nervousness:

The damn dogs prowling around always

216

cause shots during the night. Any slight noise wakes me — I must be up twenty times at night just listening.

During combat, when he wasn't on the line, his job was in the Message Center, operating phones and switchboard. The Message Center, within half a mile of the most forward troops, was exposed to fire and sneak attacks, but the rifle companies (they handled machine guns and mortars only) had it far worse.

29 May 1945

Dear, you are wrong again, your Ellery Queen deductions have led you astray. I am not a rifleman, those boys take the brunt of everything day and night, for days and weeks and months no let-up. Their job is so much harder than ours in M/C. Of course sometimes it is rough for us but nothing compares to their job.

Some days during combat, the Message Center was just a hole in the ground: "This is being written while sitting in a hole just taking telephone messages and waiting for the phone to ring." Sometimes he operated the machine "that codes and decodes our messages." He liked cryptography, "especially when the messages are tricky and I have to figure out the mistakes in them too."

He held no affection for the nights.

217

Gosh the nights are long. They are pretty rough sweating out. Every other night I'm on duty — pulling three hours on and three off. Those are the longest three hours I've ever seen. I keep thinking of ways of staying awake. Someday I may write a book on that subject. I'll write more later — it sure feels good to see morning approach.

Guard duty was shared by all the forward troops. Staying awake on your watch was crucial. The Japanese launched attacks at night. Single Japanese soldiers were hungry and desperate enough to attempt raids on U.S. supply units. The "plink plink" of pebbles falling around one's foxhole in the midnight hour could mean the beginning of a Banzai attack. Snipers were known to slip behind the lines. The danger wore at one's nerves. "We pulled guard every night in case any Nips got through the outer defenses," he wrote in July 1945, after he was in garrison and out of combat, "and in the morning we would count up the dead Nips that the boys got during the night." More than one GI had his throat slit under the cover of darkness.

Arnel swerved as a skinny dog ran across the road in front of our van. In Luzon, all breeds of dog seemed to have been reconfigured as the universal skinny dog. Dog meat is a Philippine highland delicacy, but in deference to tourist

218

sensitivities, dog carcasses were no longer on display in the Baguio open-air market.

Reading my father's letters over the past few years had deepened my understanding of the Balete campaign, but until now it had been an abstract understanding. Driving across the actual landscape fixed both the chronology of events and the strategy of combat into tactile perspective.

What was becoming physically clear at that moment, as we jounced along, was an inkling of what it meant "not to have cover." I needed to go to the bathroom. There were no trees in sight, and everywhere we looked, there were people working or walking, children playing. Arnel suggested I hang on until we reached the town of Umingan. That was the town, I remembered, where the young man from Texas, Melvin Smith, had been killed. Peter Lomenzo had described in a letter to me what it meant to an infantry soldier to have no cover:

We in the attack lay exposed in the flat rice fields. The enemy was well-entrenched with earth-fortified bunkers to house their machine guns, mortars, etc. Their rapid machine gun fire kept us pinned to the earth and amongst our casualties a platoon leader, Lt. Clark, had his face badly shot. (He did live.) And the sun just scorched our skin. We finally worked our way to the left flank into a dry river bed as our artillery (after placing a few rounds on *us*) softened them to a point where we could out-flank their protected positions and beat them off into a retreat to the next barrio where we met them again. And on and on.

The Japanese booby-trapped the bare fields and dry riverbeds with landmines. Attacking across the dry rice paddies "was like crawling across a series of pool tables; each time a soldier attempted to cross the dike separating one paddy from another, Japanese tankers, machine gunners, and riflemen laid down withering fire," Peter added.

The devastating battle for Umingan lasted until February 3, in what the official record called "hop, skip, and jump kind of warfare." The phrase sounds like a child's game, but in the battle of Umingan, U.S. GIs employed rifle grenades, bazookas, antitank guns, and fifty-caliber machine guns against the Japanese arsenal.

Somehow, during Umingan and the many hard days that followed, my father still managed to write a letter or V-mail to his wife almost every day. His buddies called him "the Ernie Pyle of the campaign" and wondered what he was writing about. His first vignettes from Luzon sometimes convey a traveler's wonder at being in a strange land.

19 January 1945
A little boy that lives in the house right near

my pup tent came up and said, "We eat now," and pointed to the house. I said, "That's a good idea. Go right ahead." But he kept repeating, "We eat now," until I realized he was inviting me into the shack to have dinner with them. I told him I wasn't hungry. This morning, a gang of kids started singing "God Bless America" until I had to tell them to please stop.

A few days later, the reality of war reappears:

Yesterday the civilians were almost frightened to death. A Jap patrol infiltrated our lines and killed some civilians and all of them started moving down the road in a stampede. The old, the young, the aged, the crippled, the sick. Mostly women and children.

The next day, his company picked up a Filipino boy who claimed to be nineteen, but looked thirteen.

He is very happy because we're going to give him a rifle and uniform. The poor kid has scars on his hands and legs from where the Japanese tortured him. He was their prisoner for a year before he escaped to the hills.

The occupying Japanese treated the Filipinos so cruelly that when the tables were turned the

Americans sometimes had to intervene: "We caught a Jap prisoner and the Filipinos wanted to cut him to pieces. We had to convince them that he was more valuable to us alive. Their attitude is the only good Nip is a dead one."

I'd learned a lot about the nature of the Japanese occupation of the Philippines from Sylvan Katz. Sylvan made it a condition of his college scholarships that his awardees go to their elders — their parents, their grandparents, older people in their barrio or town — and ask them what it was like during the war.

"I didn't ask them to write bad things about the Japanese," he told me, "but I wanted them to be aware of what happened. The old folks are dying out. There is very little said about the Japanese during the war. It's almost as if it's all forgotten — the horrible way they mistreated the people."

Sylvan sent me sheaves of these interviews. After interviewing an elder in her village, seventeen-year-old Evy Kimmayong reported: "Babies were cut out of the womb and killed with bayonets. Each woman was raped by five to ten Japanese men and after raping them the soldiers would sometimes insert a stick or an eggplant into her sex organ. Captured guerrillas were tortured, some dumped into mud, others forced to drink the water from swamps. The Japanese also forced the menfolks to rape the pigs. If they hesitated, they would be killed."

The local Filipinos, my father wrote, were "al-

222

ways eager to work for us. Dig our holes. Do our laundry. Anything at all. Mostly, they want to kill Japs. They want guns and ammunition."

More than three hundred Americans were killed at Umingan. My father's letter exhibits a chilled, subdued tone:

> 4 February 1945
> Dearest, this is the first letter to you in about a week — that is the first chance that I've had to write. I'm not going to write about combat, it isn't very pleasant. After you are in it, you don't talk about it — the sounds, smell, mud, dirt, tension, fatigue are all like a nightmare.

Miraculously, he survived the battle without a scratch, "though I might have aged a little and lost a little weight. You and Ruth were my inspiration always — whenever I was too tired to go on — and whenever I was too tired to dig a hole — I always thought of how much I have to come back to — and I'd go on. Then there is the old adage that you are caught without a hole only once."

By the tenth of February, the Central Plains phase of the Luzon Campaign was over. Some 2,654 Japanese were dead, including twenty-one-year-old Yoshio Shimizu. Three days later the troops had begun their ascent up Highway 5 toward Balete Pass. On February 13 my father reported his acquisition of Yoshio's flag. A few days later, without fanfare, he mentions, "we were all awarded the combat infantryman badge."

There's no way to know the exact circumstances of Yoshio's death, but it's fair to say he was probably spared worse to come. In the early stage of the northern Luzon Campaign, General Yamashita's troops were well fed, battle ready, convinced of their duty to kill any American rather than risk having him walk the streets of Tokyo. By the end of June, when the Twenty-fifth Infantry Division finally reached the town of Santa Fe, the downhill side of Balete Pass, Yamashita's surviving soldiers were in desperate shape — wandering around the jungle in a hallucinatory daze. They had little ammunition. They were lice-ridden. Many had malaria and other tropical diseases. Their food and medical supplies had run out. Officers ordered their soldiers to kill their own wounded comrades who could not keep moving. Early in the campaign on Balete Pass, the Japanese military command issued an order to their troops: "Positions will not be yielded to the enemy even though you die. Our only path is victory or death; therefore, defend to the last man. Those who retreat without orders will be decapitated." By June, the survivors were reduced to foraging for grains of rice in the pockets of the rags that covered their fellow soldiers' remains, or even worse — eating the flesh of their dead comrades.

In 1986, the Japanese newspaper *Asahi*

Shimbun issued a call to readers to share *their* memories of World War II. Over four thousand letters were received. One surviving Japanese veteran of Luzon described how "spending every day among dead bodies makes one doubt whether one can know where the dividing line between life and death is. One's thoughts become hazy and disorientated." That same former soldier, now a corporate executive in his seventies, also recalled his lowest moment:

> A fellow soldier whose name I didn't know came crawling over to me. Taking off his clothes, he bared his pointed rear end. It had become dark bluish-green. "Buddy, if I die, go ahead and eat this part," he said, touching his scrawny rear end with his bony finger. I said, "Idiot, how could I eat a war buddy?" But I couldn't take my eyes off the flesh on his rear.

A marauding black dog spared him the final descent into cannibalism. The man managed to fend off the beast with a knife. He stabbed it to death, roasted it, ate it with salt, and regained enough strength to stumble on.

After the Battle of Umingan, on February 10, my father sat down at a desk chair salvaged from a bombed-out schoolhouse and composed a letter. The air corps zoomed over his head, en route to a mission. He smoked his pipe and surveyed the smoldering landscape: "It would be

225

pretty if it were peaceful. But with the noise of firing and the burned out areas, and the rubble and especially the smell — God what a stench."

Half an hour past Umingan, we reached San Jose, the little town at the Highway 5 intersection. After refueling, we began to drive up mountainous Highway 5 toward Balete Pass.

The hillsides were mostly bare. Aggressive logging over the past decades has stripped away the jungle canopy. On February 21, 1945, when the Twenty-seventh Regiment was ordered to advance and secure Highway 5 from San Jose to the next little town of Digdig, these same hillsides were dense with luxuriant tropical growth: palms, clumps of bamboo, gnarled balete trees, which indigenous headhunter tribes considered sacred and never cut down.

The thick underbrush provided the Americans with plenty of cover and concealment. Unfortunately, the Japanese, who waited above them in suicidal readiness, shared the same advantage. As General Swede Larsen put it, the enemy was "looking down our throats."

Peter Lomenzo recalled, "You were always wondering about the enemy — where *was* he?" Novelist Tim O'Brien, a Vietnam vet, once commented that in Vietnam, "You couldn't *find* the enemy. So the *place* itself became the enemy." That was also true for the infantry in northern Luzon. The Japanese were dug into caves, camouflaged in bunkers. They struck at night in the dark. The place was spooky.

My father's voice sounded in my head. Why in God's name have you come to this place? Dad, I know it seems perverse. I can explain.

But I couldn't really explain. I couldn't yet answer what I hoped to learn in this place where he had spent "six long months in hell."

12 March 1945

Dearest,

I was feeling blue all day until a little while ago and this is why. We got some second-class mail and I was helping to sort them for the Battalion. I came across some mail for a fellow in our Message Center and I threw it at him.

When I walked over a little while later and glibly asked him about his hometown news, I noticed how pale and sad he was. Then he showed me the front page where one of his closest friends was killed in Europe. He couldn't snap out of it for a long while — so it had me down too.

Then along came your letters and anniversary cards and golly they gave me a lift, especially the two pictures of Ruthie. You know that's the very first picture that I have of my father since I've been overseas. The folks have never taken any snaps of themselves and I've begged them for pictures so many times. He sure looks grand. And it was a thrill seeing him and Ruthie together.

You have been writing a lot to me about my outfit, so I'll give you a bit of orientation. "Wolfhounds" is the name of our Regiment. And "Tropic Lightning" as you already know is the name of the Division. And I haven't seen any head hunters, but I've seen many other gruesome things.

Highway 5, the "national road," was a narrow strip of gravel road that hugged the side of the steep mountain. We traveled, at best, ten miles per hour. Arnel wore a grim expression. The twisting road had no shoulder, and when we encountered a truck coming from the opposite direction, we had to back around blind curves until there was a section wide enough for the truck to pass.

In 1945, when my father was here, this entire rugged area was unmapped. The army gave names to strategic sites: Norton's Knob, the Wart, Lone Tree Hill, Wolfhouse Ridge — each one the locus of a ferocious engagement with the Japanese. The terrain, even now, was incredibly rough.

Yamashita's troops contested every step of the Twenty-fifth Division's advance toward Balete Pass. They honeycombed the ridges with a maze of tunnels and caves, some as long as forty feet. Yamashita's tragic error, states the *U.S. Army in World War II*, "was in not anticipating the cave-sealing technique devised by 25th Division troops."

Into the caves they threw explosives, white phosphorus bombs, flamethrowers — incinerating the occupants. Sometimes Japanese soldiers ran out, their clothes on fire. Then they were shot down. "You had to stay to the side before you threw anything in, so they couldn't shoot you," Sylvan Katz recalled. He also remembered the time his unit took a position on a ridge for eight days, directly above a sealed Japanese cave. "I was standing with another GI, a guy we called 'the minister' (he'd been to divinity school) and we were talking. We noticed that the ground underneath us was moving, then it opened. An emaciated Japanese soldier emerged from the hole. He was nearly naked. His only tool was a U.S. Army spoon. He'd been in the dark for around five or six days, because we were in our positions that long. It took him all that time to dig his way out." I gasped. "The minister shot him," said Sylvan. "No questions asked."

Another factor Yamashita couldn't have foreseen: tanks. With much ingenuity and great effort, engineers from the Twenty-fifth managed to get tanks up the mountains. The tanks moved along ridges so narrow that portions of their treads hung over the edge. The Japanese had not brought any antitank weapons up with them from the Central Plains into the mountains. They never imagined the Americans would be able to bring tanks up the precipitous heights. According to the *U.S. Army in World War II*,

"Many Japanese, overcome by surprise as tanks loomed up through the forest, abandoned their prepared defenses and fled."

As we wound higher and higher up the slopes, I tried not to look down. Large sections of road simply weren't there — washed out by the last typhoon or cracked off the side of the mountain by an earthquake. Occasionally we passed work crews, barefoot men with trowels, repairing a section of road; it looked to be an interminable project. As soon as they repaired one section, Mother Nature ruined it again.

Peter Lomenzo was the Twenty-seventh Infantry Regiment's staff officer during the battle for Balete Pass. His job, "under the colonel's name" as he describes it, was to lay out the plan for attack. "To understand the battle for Balete Pass," he told me, "you have to keep in mind the most salient fact: *It was uphill,* so you were always tired. Tired beyond imagination. You were always struggling against fatigue." Army uniforms are called fatigues for a reason.

My father's fatigue persisted for years after the war ended. It was Balete Pass that did it; those 165 days of fear and uphill stress wore him out. Combat, the aftermath of combat, and the anticipation of combat all wear you down. Months of continuous combat, continual fight-or-flight arousal conditions, take the human body's nervous system to its furthest extremes. It's not uncommon for a soldier in combat to urinate or defecate in his pants. The body, literally "blows

230

its ballast." The physiological price for this constant revving of the nervous system — in its aftermath, an incredibly powerful weariness.

I can still see my father's frame sunk into his armchair, asleep after dinner, night after night, for so many years after the war. I still hear in my head that repeated phrase, "Don't wake your father, he's so tired." He was perpetually fatigued.

On March 17, the Twenty-seventh Regiment began an attack some three thousand yards south of Balete Pass where the Japanese had organized their main line of resistance. The underbrush was so dense, they had to cover some of the distance on hands and knees. The Twenty-fifth Division yearbook describes "torturous, close-in fighting." The Americans were then less than five miles from the pass. But it would take two months to cover that distance.

24 April 1945

Dearest,
I can honestly say that the last three weeks have been the most miserable, unhappiest, gruesomest, most fatiguing that I have ever lived through. And the worst of it is that it isn't over yet. Tomorrow I have to go back to it.

In a way, I'm glad that I didn't write. I would have written in a very despairing and morbid style.

It's a wonder that I didn't come down

231

with some illness, for several days I slept in mud and was so cold I couldn't stop shivering — my body and hands, and teeth just were uncontrollable.

I've just been thinking for awhile. It's hard to realize that I've been sleeping on the ground and in holes for over a hundred days now. I've seen sights and lived through things that have left an indelible impression on my mind. This damn campaign can't go on forever. We're bound to get a break some day.

As his comrades "went the way of Dr. Orange," my father referred to combat as the "Buzz Saw of War." Others called it "the meat grinder" because of the way war in this tropical hell devoured men. He warned my mother, "I'm going to be a pretty hard guy when I get back — this army really has toughened me. I don't take any crap from anyone — and everyone really respects me for it."

Arnel maneuvered the van up the precarious pitted road toward the three-thousand-foot summit of Balete Pass. The van's heat gauge pegged past the neutral zone. Arnel snapped off the air conditioner. The ninety-degree-plus heat made me dopey. We'd been traveling since morning, and it was nearly three o'clock in the afternoon.

Just when I could see ahead where the grade

leveled off, the left rear of the van gave a threatening hiss, then sighed and sank. Flat tire. Arnel managed to get the van to a pull-off, then pointed toward a klatch of small buildings up the road. Maybe someone there could give him a hand.

We scrambled out. As Arnel pulled out of sight, we looked around and noticed a curious concrete column across the road. As we walked toward it, we saw that it was the marker constructed by the Twenty-fifth Infantry in May 1945 to commemorate the Balete Pass Campaign.

On May 10, the Wolfhounds finally declared Balete Pass secure. "Thus," it is recorded in the Twenty-fifth Infantry yearbook, "the operation from San Jose to the strategic 'front door to the Cagayan Valley' — 33 miles of bitter, yard-by-yard fighting — had reached its climax." Lieutenant Peter Lomenzo remembers making a radio call to Colonel Lindeman, his commanding officer, to assure him that his men were indeed at Balete Pass: "I told him that I was pissing on it and could see the other side."

The commemorative column was far less grand than it looked in the Twenty-fifth Division yearbook. No longer was the approach set up on a walkway of mortared stone. It was low on the ground and dwarfed by a nearby radio antenna as well as a monument to victims of the latest typhoon.

The plaque on the column read:

ERECTED IN
HONOR OF THOSE
SOLDIERS OF THE
25TH DIVISION WHO
SACRIFICED THEIR
LIVES IN WINNING
THIS DESPERATE
STRUGGLE
BALETE PASS

IN TAKING THIS PASS 7403 JAPS
COUNTED KILLED
2365 25TH DIV. KILLED & WOUNDED
MAY 13, 1945

General MacArthur announced to the press on May 15, 1945, that Balete Pass had been won. However, numerous American casualties — including the loss of General Dalton on May 16 and Sam Wengrow later that same month — occurred during the fierce "mop up," which lasted until June 30. By then, the final toll of Japanese known dead during the entire Luzon Campaign would be 14,569 — with 614 taken prisoner. On September 2, 1945, the same day Japan surrendered to the Allies, General Yamashita and his staff officers walked out of the Caraballo Mountains and surrendered.

Filipino litter-bearers had carried out the American wounded and dead. I asked Sylvan Katz if the Japanese dead had been buried up at Balete Pass, another question that exposed my naivete. "We weren't about to risk our men to carry out their dead," he said patiently.

In Los Angeles, I interviewed a woman from the Philippines named Salud Ilao, who'd been a nurse's aide for the Twenty-fifth Division near Balete Pass. She remembered it differently: "As soon as a battle was over, the American engineers cleared away the bodies, buried them in a hole. It was because of sanitation."

A bit of both is probably true. Sometimes the American engineers would bulldoze the bodies of the enemy dead into mass graves. Because the flanks of Balete Pass were so steep, bulldozers were in short supply. The Japanese dead littered the landscape. Or they died alone of starvation in jungle-choked ravines. The wounded, who asked their medics for painkillers, were more likely given a grenade to blow themselves up. Unknown thousands of Japanese soldiers had been sealed into caves and dugouts surrounding Balete Pass.

Most of the Japanese dead suffered the fate soldiers fear the most — their flesh reduced to meat. In Homer's *Iliad*, a soldier who died unburied was considered doubly defeated — first by the enemy and then by the scavenging buzzards and dogs who clean up the battlefield when the fight is over.

In *The Burmese Harp*, Kon Ichikawa's powerful 1956 antiwar film, a Japanese infantryman realizes the purposelessness of war and is transformed by his realization. He takes the vows of a

Buddhist monk and dedicates his life to collecting and burying the remains of his dead comrades whose corpses litter the landscape of war-ravaged Burma. It's a poignant fiction. In reality, the bodies of Yoshio Shimizu and his dead comrades probably decomposed in trenches in the open fields around Umingan, or in caves sealed into the brushy slopes of the Caraballo Mountains.

We walked past the Balete Pass marker to the concrete typhoon monument. There was a small door on the side. We entered and climbed up a spiral staircase. The stairwell was stiflingly hot and filled with trash.

From the top I could see down the other side of the pass, toward rice-terraced hills, which were, as Peter Lomenzo recalled, "as green as Ireland." Glancing up, Lloyd caught sight of a cluster of larger structures farther up the hill. "Maybe they've built another monument to the Twenty-fifth Division," he suggested.

We trudged up the hill. The path leveled out on the plateau, where there was an open area ringed by at least five mammoth dark-gray granite markers. I started to read the plaque on the nearest one, and for a few moments wondered why I couldn't decipher the writing. Then I realized: The writing was in Japanese. These were all monuments erected after the war by the Japanese.

One plaque had an English translation: It

spoke of "universal peace," of the eternal rest of all the soldiers — American, Filipino, Japanese — who had died at Balete Pass. The irony was superb: After losing this ferocious battle to the Americans, who struggled uphill for more than a hundred days, the Japanese had claimed the higher ground.

I was shocked by the unpeaceful feelings surging through me. I felt my father's anger erupt in my own body.

A calmer voice intruded. More than sixteen thousand souls were floating around Balete Pass. More Japanese than Americans died here. What would all those dead have to say? What would Sam Wengrow, lying in a grave in the American Cemetery in Manila, have to say about this place, this war? Had *he* forgiven his enemies? Had he met Yoshio on the other side? Did Yoshio believe in the emperor's war at the moment of his death?

"I know you have a certain empathy for the flag-bearing Japanese soldier," Peter Lomenzo had once written me. "I understand that. But believe me (and I fought in three major campaigns and innumerable battles) — the Japanese enemy was just that in *every sense* of the word." When Sylvan had told me about the soldier who'd dug his way out of a tunnel with an Army spoon, I'd asked, "Didn't you think he wanted to surrender?" He'd replied without sentiment, "He was just a Japanese soldier."

The image of the Shimizus outside the window of my train compartment returned to me. Spirits of ancestors and offspring — of those who died and those who survived — commingled on this steep, scrubby mountain pass.

I couldn't expect my combat veteran friends to forgive. That would have to be left to future generations. At least we could try to understand what all these men had gone through, bear witness to their suffering. *That,* I realized, was why I was here.

In spite of the oppressive afternoon heat, I started to shiver. Lloyd gripped my shoulder. We walked down the hill to the highway and headed in the direction we'd last seen Arnel and the van. Across the road, three young boys in ragged T-shirts yelled, "Hey you! Rich Americans! Give us dollars! We're so poor!" Lloyd returned their yells and gestured them toward us.

Arnel and the van lumbered up the steep incline. He pulled over to the side of the road and got out. Followed by our three new friends, we all walked over to a tiny kitchen under a palapa by the side of the road. Three little tables with plastic checkered tablecloths, a framed portrait of the Virgin Mary graced the stained stucco wall. The aproned matron who took our order had a hand-rolled cigarette dangling from her lips. A plastic flyswatter was tucked in her waistband. The two young men who had helped Arnel change a tire also joined us. We ordered cold Coca-Colas and platefuls of sliced mangoes.

While everyone ate and drank, I imagined an eerie brigade of shades, black dogs growling at their heels, trooping sorrowfully over these hills. I was grateful for the laughter of the living, grateful to return to the present.

It was well after midnight when we returned to Baguio. Lloyd and I crept into our room at the inn and slid, exhausted, under the cotton sheets. From the Sound and Motion Western Ballroom on the street behind the inn, the evening's entertainer crooned lyrics about hard luck, the vagaries of troubled love.

I pressed closer to Lloyd and thought of a tender passage from one of my dad's letters to my mother:

> After months of dreading nighttime, especially a night too bright or too dark, it is so hard to change. So you see that I need you to help me get over that type of fear and use the nights for what they were meant for.

I wept for my dead father. I wept for Sam Wengrow lying in the American Cemetery, and for Melvin Smith, who died in Umingan. I wept for all those souls haunting Balete Pass. And, yes, I wept for Yoshio Shimizu, who never made it home to Suibara.

Then together, my husband and I used the night for what it was meant for.

CHAPTER FOURTEEN

Promised Land

On the very last day of 1945, my parents heard each other's voices for the first time in over two full years. The next morning, my father recorded his reactions in the same way he had done almost every day during that separation: he wrote a letter home.

> Vancouver Barracks —
> Vancouver, Washington
> 31 December 1945

My Dearest,
The writing habit is so very strong after these many months of corresponding that I'm just compelled to sit down and write to you. Mostly though, I'm just so very lonesome for you.

Last night when we spoke on the phone after two full years, I was in a daze — as though I were dreaming all this. When I spoke to my mother, she was so excited and almost screamed into the phone. I could hardly talk. That was when your call came through. I was more composed by then.

It sure was a wonderful coincidence to have Ruthie awake and on your lap just as that time in the early morning when the call finally did come to you.

I may have to get a discharge in Fort Mac-Arthur because there was no other way out if I were to stop and see the folks first in L.A. But that is the Army and anyway, the cost to go cross-country isn't all the money in the world.

It's been two long years, Dearest. I had hoped to be with you for this Christmas and New Year's but Time, Fate, and this Damn Army —

Anyway my slogan of "Home Alive in '45" came true. See you soon. I'll call you again before you get this letter. I love you — Norman

It was the 474th letter he'd written since leaving for the Pacific front — and the last. After this letter, my father left no record of how he felt from day to day — no record of what he did, what he read, to whom he spoke. Writing letters had been his way of bridging distance. After the war, there was no longer any physical distance to bridge; my father lived a mostly sedentary life. Given a choice, he preferred to stay home.

As we returned home from the Philippines, I began to wonder what it had been like for my father to begin life over again. California had been his promised land during the war — if he could just make it through, back to my mother, then they would be able to build a new life together.

I thought of a story my mother told me about my father not long before she died. It was March 1946. The war was over. Hiroshima was in ruins. On Sycamore Street, in a quiet neighborhood in the heart of Los Angeles where they had recently settled, the young couple who were not yet my father and mother strolled hand in hand. Recently reunited, these two were in love.

Leafy sycamore branches cast mottled shadows on the sidewalk. Tawny trunks, new bark peeking out under patches of the old, reflected the glaring southern California light. The street was lined with solid duplexes and triplexes in a variety of architectural styles: red-roofed Spanish, Moorish fantasy, French chateau, faux Rococo. Inside those apartments on Sycamore Street, housewives ironed, clipped grocery coupons from the newspaper, heated formula, set macaroni and cheese on the table.

My father, then thirty, was still lean and muscular from combat in the Philippines, but he walked with the slow deliberate step of the stockier, softer man he would later become. His army buzz cut had grown out and his blue-black hair waved upward from his brow like Van Cliburn's. His young blue-eyed wife wore her bangs short across her forehead. Her step was more exuberant, but she restrained herself in deference to her husband's more dignified pace.

My father had waited two and a half years for this: to walk down a safe sun-dappled street in civilian clothes, holding his wife's hand. The long separation — the jungle fighting, foxholes, bloated corpses — was only a nightmare. My father was determined to forget all that, or at least that's what he claimed.

On that late afternoon in the early spring of 1946, he pulled his wife closer to him, inhaling the sweet smell of her hair. As they approached the corner of Sycamore Street and Beverly Boulevard, he noticed a trim soldier emerge from the canopied walkway of the most elegant apartment building on the block. Not just any soldier, but a soldier wearing the distinctive shoulder patch of the Twenty-fifth Infantry Division: a red taro leaf emblazoned with a yellow zigzag, the insignia of "Tropic Lightning."

Without hesitation, he dropped his wife's hand and sprinted toward his presumed comrade. In his rush, he failed to notice the cables, the klieg lights, the director's chair. Before he could reach the handsome soldier, two burly security guards lunged forward and tackled him to the ground. Their job was to prevent reality from intruding on illusion.

Dazed, he lay on his back looking upward through sycamore leaves toward blue sky. "Who the hell are you?" growled one of the security guards. "Norman Steinman," my father sputtered back, gesturing toward the uniformed soldier. "I was just demobbed from that outfit."

The guard stepped aside and my father now looked up into the anxious face of the man he'd been racing to embrace. "Let him go!" the soldier admonished, extending his hand. Warily, my father grasped the proffered hand and allowed himself to be pulled to his feet. Only then, looking the man square in the face, did he recognize the actor Frederic March. My father, the just-returned GI, had stumbled upon the set of William Wyler's *The Best Years of Our Lives*, what would become the classic American film of GIs returning home from World War II.

My mother, in her high heels, was still four houses from the corner when she saw him go down. Arriving on the scene, she watched in astonishment as her favorite leading man dusted off her husband's gabardine slacks. Frederic March offered him a crisp salute as the grips and gaffers cheered. "You must forgive me," he said in a grave tone of apology. "I'm just a powder-puff soldier."

Frederic March had not spent nights shivering in his foxhole. He had not buried his buddies, or walked for days in wet boots, or watched kamikaze pilots fall from the sky in brilliant clouds of fire. He was right to offer apologies to my father for the indignity of being tackled to the ground.

I've watched Wyler's film many times by now. There's one scene that always holds my attention: the first morning home for Sergeant Al Stevenson (Frederic March) after three years of combat in the Pacific. Still in his pajamas, Al sinks into his favorite armchair and rests his feet on a hassock. He's not yet at ease in the lap of comfort. How can his loving wife and children who gather around him possibly imagine what Dad's been through "over there"? Next to Al's chair is his worn army duffel. He reaches into it and pulls out a three-foot-long Japanese samurai sword. Without saying a word, he unsheathes it from its scabbard and hands it to his bewildered teenage son.

The war hero reaches into his duffel bag a second time and pulls out a Japanese flag with characters written all over it. "I got it off a dead Jap," he says brightly. "The writings on it are messages of good luck from the soldier's family and friends." He offers this also to his son, who handles it cautiously, as if it were contaminated.

Al Stevenson has a daughter as well, but he does not consider offering his war trophies to her. Perhaps he brought her a kimono or a doll, but the distribution of the *real* spoils of war are usually patrilineal. War is considered the province of men and, just as mothers presumably share the secrets of childbirth with their grown daughters, it is a father's prerogative to tell his son about his experiences in war.

Just before they were shipped home from occupied Japan in November 1945, the Twenty-fifth Division drew war trophies. My father wrote that he'd received "a fairly nice saber. Very good blade and mediocre scabbard and handle — but I'm satisfied." He had no intention of bequeathing the sword to his still-infant daughter. "You're probably thinking now what on earth are we going to do with it — another thing to keep out of little Ruthie's way. Well it's just like any other trophy — just to hang over the mantelpiece — or show to our son many years hence."

When we were children, when our parents weren't home, my older brother, Larry, and I dared each other to take the sword out of the closet. We crawled underneath the soft hems of our mother's rayon dresses to excavate the heavy metal shaft from its obscure corner.

Larry drew the sword out of its scabbard. Through the louvered windows of our parents' bedroom, turquoise light shimmered off the surface of the swimming pool, illuminating the fine Japanese steel. We lightly ran our fingertips over the golden chrysanthemum embossed on the hilt. We carefully tested the edge of the razor-sharp blade.

My father was always planning to have a son, and in time, he was blessed with two. He intended to give his first son the saber, but he never did. He kept it hidden away in the back of his closet for fifty years.

As for Yoshio's flag with the black-inked calligraphy and the rust-red speckles? He never intended to bequeath that to anyone.

PART IV

Suibara

CHAPTER FIFTEEN

Swans in the Morning

I tiptoe across the lobby, dimly lit by fluorescent vending machines. I'm the first guest up. At the front desk, the gap-toothed night watchman obligingly hands me binoculars. "Hakchyo?" he asks. "Swans?" I nod vigorously. Yes, 4,658 of them by yesterday's posted count. I step into my boots, pull down my earflaps, and head outside into steady snow.

It's December 1998 and I've returned to Suibara. Since our brief visit three years ago, I'd been yearning to see the Shimizus again, to deepen my understanding of what life was like in Yoshio's town before, during, and after the war. And of course, I remembered the Swan Uncle's invitation — to see Lake Hyoko during swan season. On this trip, with Lloyd working on a project in Los Angeles, I have traveled alone.

Outside, in the predawn dimness, I walk away from the inn and into a medieval landscape painting: pure white swans rousing themselves on an ice-fringed lake. Lake Hyoko reverberates with a glorious dissonance. The morning greetings of thousands of whooper swans — plus assorted mallards, widgeons, teals, and grebes — sound like a hundred orchestras tuning up simultaneously in the same concert hall. Sunlight leaks over the nearby Ise mountain range. The mighty five-foot-tall birds begin their takeoff, actually "running" on the water to gain enough speed to lift their heavy bodies into the air. It's a thrilling spectacle: thousands of birds rising en masse then skimming over the lake toward the sun.

Before coming to Suibara, I met with Masako. We'd been corresponding these past few years and by now we felt like old friends. She had continued to be the go-between between the Shimizus and me, ferrying messages and gifts. "I called the Shimizus to tell them you were coming, I spoke to Suezo," she said. "He told me, 'I just dreamed of Louise-san last night.' As if he were expecting you."

The mayor's office in Suibara has established an ambitious schedule for my week-long stay. They have contacted a number of Suibara villagers who are war veterans or have memories of the war years in Suibara and are willing to speak with me. There also will be a gathering at Suezo's house. Masako has generously offered to travel every day from her home in Nagaoka to be the translator during these meetings.

Mr. Mihara, the mayor's energetic young assistant, meets us at the Suibara train station and we drive to the town's first guest house, the

Rhythm Inn. Puzzled, I ask Masako, "Why 'Rhythm'?" "From tou*r-ism*," she shrugs, laughing.

The banner over the front door reads "Welcome, Mrs. Steinman." The manager, an officious man in a black suit and tie, rushes out to greet me. I am his first American guest. Though Suibara draws Japanese tourists in the winter swan season, it's not exactly a mecca for Westerners. After Masako and Mr. Mihara leave, there's no one around who speaks English, but the staff is friendly and we communicate through sign language and giggles.

Each afternoon, Masako and Mr. Mihara pick me up in the city van and we drive to the cultural center. In a bare white classroom, buoyed by cans of hot green tea, we meet our interviewees. Speaking to someone you have just met, across a table, with a translator, is an inherently formal situation. Yet in all these interviews, there is the desire, on both sides, to transcend the limitations.

Our first guests are Mrs. Seito, an eighty-six-year-old farmwife, and Mrs. Nakayama, an eighty-eight-year-old former second-grade teacher. Both women were widowed during the war; they have outlived their husbands by more than fifty years. Seito-san has a wide face crisscrossed with well-earned wrinkles; her smile reveals a mouthful of crooked gold and silver teeth. Nakayama-sensei ("teacher") is more regal, finer-boned than Mrs. Seito, though hobbled by arthritis.

Mrs. Nakayama's husband, Takeo, was drafted October 1, 1943, and died December 29 that same year, in Java. She learned of his death two years later. "When he died, I had two children and my mother-in-law to care for. I had a teaching job. We had to eat potato leaves, potato stems." War widows did not have it easy; Japanese culture is traditionally unkind to women without men.

"Pearl Harbor Day was a day just like today," Mrs. Seito remarks, "it snowed all day." She glances out the window of the classroom at an overcast sky, snow dusting the bare branches of a persimmon tree. Mrs. Seito's husband, Hideo, was drafted in 1942 at the age of twenty-two. His submarine was sunk by a torpedo en route from Manila to Burma, in 1944. Three years later, his family received an official announcement. "I still have the envelope," she sighs. "In those days we were told that Japan was doing the right thing, and the United States was our enemy. That's what we were told. But I never thought we could fight against Americans. I thought a country called America was a far-off place filled with rich, strong, very clever people."

Eventually, the government sent her a box purporting to contain her husband's bones. "I was suspicious," she says, "how could they have found his bones if he'd drowned at sea?" She opened the box and found dry twigs.

More than one bereaved woman told me there

was a moment when she intuited her husband's — or son's or brother's — death. There were omens: a bowl inexplicably breaking, a dog's melancholy howling piercing the silence of a snowy night. Mrs. Seito says, "There was some strange cracking sound near the portable shrine in my house. We went to look around the room, but nothing had happened. That was the time that my husband died."

From the two widows, I learn how, during World War II, the military siphoned off Suibara's agricultural bounty. The storerooms of rice, the barrels of miso and soy, the mounds of huge green cabbages, the bushels of white daikon — all were requisitioned. "We had to give all the rice harvest to the government, even though we had nothing," Mrs. Seito tells me. The people of Suibara ate tree bark and foraged in the mountains for wild greens. "You saw how a person could 'grow thin like a mantis.'" Suibara schoolchildren were dismissed from school to collect sap from the pines in the mountain foothills, part of a military scheme to make ersatz fuel for what was left of Japan's air fleet. Farmers watched anxiously overhead for American B-29s while tilling their fields and, in an era of virulent nationalism, watched their tongues lest the dreaded Kempetai (military police) suspect them of any unpatriotic utterances.

In the summer of 1945, the villagers began training for the ultimate battle, the American invasion of the mainland. Suibara villagers sharpened bamboo "spears" and practiced using them on bales of hay under the eyes of retired soldiers. Even though official propaganda concealed most news of Japan's defeats in the Pacific, many suspected their efforts would be useless against the weaponry of such a powerful foe.

Mrs. Seito was summoned by her neighborhood chief to listen to the emperor's historic surrender speech on August 15, 1945. Static obscured much of what the emperor uttered in a quivery voice. "But when we realized that Japan had surrendered," Mrs. Seito recalls, "all the energy went out of our bodies. We became weak, exhausted." *Shikata ga nai.* What could they do? They had to reconstruct their town, their country, their lives.

On New Year's Day 1946, the emperor made another radio address to the nation, and, in a speech written by an advisor to General MacArthur, renounced his divinity. As the writer Ian Buruma has noted, "It was, perhaps, the first time in human history that God had to declare himself dead." Later that spring, Suibara's men who'd survived the war began to arrive home.

Isamu Watanabe, a handsome, silver-haired seventy-four-year-old man and former mayor of Suibara, was an army private on Japan's southernmost island of Shikoku, where he'd been digging "octopus holes" along the coastline. Japanese soldiers were supposed to conceal themselves in these holes when the Americans invaded. From a distance of 150 kilometers, he'd seen the cloud from the bomb dropped on Hiroshima. En route home to Suibara, he stopped in the ruined city to see for himself the extent of the devastation. Mr. Watanabe also made a stop in Niigata, where he saw bone-thin American POWs who'd barely survived the war.

"People criticized young men if they didn't join the army," he says, "and the training was very very strict." He touches his cheek where, he tells me, officers slapped recruits with their leather slippers. "We were educated from very young that we must fight against our enemies. Soldiers were told to say, 'Heil emperor! Banzai!' when they died, but in reality, no one said that, they all cried for their mothers."

My father, I tell him, could never talk about the war. "I understand that," he responds thoughtfully. "Many Japanese soldiers could not talk about it either, because it was so cruel."

Mr. Watanabe picks up a piece of chalk and draws a crude timeline on the blackboard. He marks off the prehistoric Jomon period; the Edo era, when the feudal Shibata clan built Lake Hyoko as a reservoir; Commodore Perry's arrival in Japan in 1853; the Meiji Restoration that followed; the Manchurian Incident of 1931; Pearl Harbor, December 7, 1941; and January 1945, when Yoshio died in Luzon. His timeline ends on April 15, 1995, "when Yoshio Shimizu's flag came home." He wipes the dust chalk off his hands and sits down.

In 1947, Emperor Hirohito himself passed

through Suibara, an orchestrated countrywide tour intended to humanize the "divine" emperor by having him personally greet his subjects. What most Suibarans remember seeing of him was the top of his gray fedora. That same year, Mrs. Nakayama, the teacher, joined one of the many volunteer brigades that journeyed to Tokyo to rake leaves and repair the gardens of the emperor's Imperial Palace. She remembers the great numbers of orphaned children wandering around Tokyo, sleeping under bombed-out bridges, scavenging for cigarette butts and scraps of food.

"One day in the barbershop I was very shocked and sad to hear a young man say that the war dead were very stupid people," Mrs. Nakayama comments. "He said only stupid people died. It is quite difficult to tell the young people what the war was like, for them to understand what we went through."

Young people I spoke to in Japan knew little about their elders' experiences in the war. In the collection of letters about the war written to the newspaper *Asahi Shimbun* was one from a thirty-one-year-old housewife named Kishida Mayumi. She had never once heard her father speak of his wartime experiences. All she had learned from her mother was that her father had gone to Manchuria as an army soldier, and that he had returned with an orphaned girl and three children of relatives who had died. She noticed that when by chance a Chinese person spoke to her father, he answered in Chinese. "I wondered what Father had seen and what he had done. I have no way of asking him now. But I wonder if his refusal to accept his military pension and his repudiation of those who sang military songs were Father's way of expressing how he felt about the War — the war that Father never spoke a word about. What Father taught me about the War was the scar from a bullet passing though his thigh and the heavy, gruesome pain residing in his heart."

In his book, *Embracing Defeat: Japan in the Wake of World War II*, John Dower describes the moral and psychological dilemma facing families like the Shimizus, widows like Mrs. Seito and Mrs. Nakayama, and former soldiers who'd lost friends in combat after the surrender: What do you tell the dead when you lose a war? That they were deceived? That their deaths didn't mean anything?

In Japan, one universally accepted way to mourn the war dead is to be a proponent of peace. A major tenet of the Japanese peace movement, Dower points out, is "to champion a nonmilitarized, nonnuclearized world." Without exception, everyone I spoke to in Suibara and elsewhere in Japan professed their abhorrence for war, their gratitude for peace.

Over the five years following Japan's surrender, soldiers from Suibara who'd served in Manchuria, or on the Korea-Chinese border, returned from prison camps in Russia and

257

China. Mr. Abe, eighty-four, a former hospital administrator, spent four years in a Siberian prison camp after just one week of active service in Korea. Mr. Abe, slight but powerfully built, is also a judo master. "When I was captured by the Russians, I never expected to see Japan again," he says flatly. His family presumed he was dead. I ask cautiously, "Can you tell me what your life in the camp was like?" Mr. Abe does not respond at first, then he emits a quiet groan. "I didn't want to tell you because I didn't want to remember — but I *will* tell you."

He describes some basics of prison life in Stalin's Russia: little food beyond black bread and water, bitter cold, hard labor in a lumber mill and on construction sites. "What gave you the strength to survive?" I ask. "My strong desire to go back to Japan, to home," he replies. "I was very young. I didn't want to die in such a terrible place. Also, I have practiced judo since I was thirteen, so I had this strong wish not to be defeated."

Russian citizens who were not prisoners worked alongside the Japanese POWs on construction sites. Mr. Abe learned some Russian and they conversed. "I found them quite open-minded," he says. "We didn't feel that those people were our enemies. I feel that war broke out between the higher-ranking government officials, politicians — not between ordinary people." He thinks Japan should apologize for its depredations in Asia to the Koreans and to the

Chinese. "It is the right thing to do," he says firmly. Then he sighs. "But apologies are the hardest thing for human beings to do."

In 1949, when he was finally repatriated, Mr. Abe's family learned he was still alive, and Mr. Abe learned his father had just died. Five hundred and seventy-four of Suibara's young men perished in *Dai Towa Senso,* "The Greater East Asia War," as World War II is known in Japan. More would never be accounted for. The town, Mr. Abe says, "was unrecognizable. Everything was in disrepair. And the people's minds were not at peace."

We pull out of the parking lot of the community center, winding through the narrow streets of Suibara's central shopping district. Santa Claus cutouts decorate store windows and an ultracheery "Jingle Bells" trickles out from speakers mounted on street lamps. Mr. Mihara stops the van in front of an old rickety wooden building. "Come," he says, "I want to show you something."

The huge building was once a junior high school. I peer through cracks in boarded-up windows: inside, a rusted woodstove, the remnants of a blackboard, chairs and desks.

"Yoshio went to school here?"

Mihara-san nods.

On a lot behind the old school, a new building is under construction. I laugh as Mr. Mihara strikes an odd pose, standing on one leg with his arms outstretched behind him. He's showing me the architectural design of the new school, which mimics a swan in flight.

That night at the Rhythm Inn, I stay up late, waiting until everyone has taken their bath so I can take mine in private. Many villagers come in the evening to bathe with their children in the communal bath.

Near eleven P.M., too tired to wait any longer, I overcome my shyness and pad through the lobby in my slippers and yukata (robe) toward the women's side of the communal bathing area. I place my robe and slippers in a wicker basket in the changing room and push open the door leading to the tub. A grandmother, her grown daughter, and her two-year-old granddaughter are immersed in the sunken tiled bath. As my guidebook instructs, I squat on a plastic stool under a shower faucet to wash and rinse before entering the tub. Then, self-conscious, I ease myself into the blissfully hot water.

The two women smile at me. The young mother is pearly white with pendulous breasts; her daughter, whom the grandmother scrubs energetically, is plump and rosy. I can't help but notice the sculpted curves of these three generations, their comfort with their own bodies, with the water, with each other.

My tight muscles and tired mind give way in the moist heat. So many unknowables in a life, I think dreamily. Unknowables mixed with miracles. My father's sister dying young of a tiny hole in her heart. Five thousand Siberian swans on a snowy lake. My mother hearing my father's voice after two years' separation. How a name on a piece of cloth could propel you halfway around the world.

The baby girl splashes water at me; I startle out of my reverie and we all laugh. In Japan, I now realize, half the experience of bathing is sharing the bath with others. I love being here, naked and at ease with these women on this wintry night in Suibara.

The next day, Masako, Mr. Mihara, and I drive to Suezo Shimizu's house. Across the road from the house, a neighbor's funeral is in progress. Elaborate floral wreaths brighten the weathered gray boards of the garage where a hearse idles. Black-robed Buddhist priests clang bells. Mourners mill about on the soggy grass; some hold bags of sugar, for reasons I never remember to find out.

At their door, the Shimizus greet me with great warmth. Suezo looks frailer now than he did three years ago. He squeezes my hand heartily and inquires after Lloyd. Yoshinobu, his nephew, is there with three daughters in tow, two new babies since I last visited. The three Shimizu sisters — Hanayo, Hiroshi, Chiyono — all join us at the long table in the tatami room, as well as cousin Yasue Shimizu and four childhood friends of Yoshio Shimizu — Hisashi, Yukio, Tatue, and Tokue — plus assorted neighbors. I notice Yoshio's flag, now framed and behind glass, in a special alcove in the corner.

After introductions all around, the party breaks into smaller convivial groups. The women huddle at one end of the table, talking and laughing. I sit with the men, the war veterans, who drink beer and swap stories. Yoshio Shimizu's childhood friends reminisce — how Yoshio used to play hooky from school ("but always told the truth about it"), how they all played war games together. They tell me that like so many young boys eager to escape the farmer's harsh life for the romantic adventure of military living, Yoshio enlisted. *He wanted to go.* I hadn't imagined it that way.

The funeral procession next door is about to depart. I join the Shimizu family in their front yard to pay respects to the deceased — an eighty-eight-year-old grandmother. Somehow, it feels right to be standing as part of this family, bowing together with them as the hearse drives out of the narrow alley. Hiroshi Shimizu sprinkles salt on me before I reenter the house, a custom not unlike the Jewish tradition of washing your hands after visiting a cemetery.

Back inside, we reassemble at the table and continue eating and talking. I learn from Suezo that in the war the Shimizu family lost not one but *three* sons: Heijiro, Yomatsu, and Yoshio.

Two shy young girls enter the room, carrying their English textbooks. They want to practice

262

speaking English with me. Suezo asks me to explain to his young niece and her friend the story of the flag. With Masako's occasional intervention, I do. Suezo watches us, pleased. The two girls listen, eyes wide. They're trying to make sense of how this flag has brought an American woman from Los Angeles to eat lunch in their great-uncle's living room.

Together, I realize, we are creating a new transfamilial history. At Passover a year ago, my own siblings and niece and nephews gathered in Palo Alto, where as part of the holiday text, my brother Larry read aloud a poem I had written about the flag of Yoshio Shimizu. Through a traumatic encounter on a battlefield, our families — Steinman and Shimizu — share a story. Each family will continue to tell it in their own way.

When it's time to leave, Suezo bows and offers a warm hand to say good-bye. This is probably the last time I'll see the elder Shimizus. Masako translates Suezo's softly uttered parting words: "You have given us back Yoshio. The government only sent sand in a box."

CHAPTER SIXTEEN

Flyover

Before dawn, I walk around the gourd-shaped lake. I stop in front of the bronze statue of Jusaburo Yoshikawa, the farmer whose love and perseverance ultimately made the swans feel welcome on Lake Hyoko. "It won't do to just watch the swans and feed them," the Swan Father used to admonish the villagers. "You must become a swan yourself."

Several swan duets are in progress this morning — heads thrust forward and back in rhythmic sequences, there's much wing-flapping and preening.

As the day brightens and the flock lifts off, I turn down a road in the direction of the mountains, past fine old two-story farmhouses with blue-tiled roofs. The farmers have clothed their fruit trees and shrubs with "coats" of twine and bamboo sticks; some are provided with their own umbrellas, to lessen the weight of snow on their branches. Neat rows of taro and kale stretch out into the distance. Strings of daikon, garlic, onions, and lotus root dry on racks hanging from barn eaves. A woman rinses a bucket of rags in an irrigation canal. There are few people around, and no one pays me much attention.

I pass a room-size wooden shrine in the middle of a small cedar grove. The gate opens easily; I walk in. At the edge of the copse, I stare out at a rice paddy where a few swans glean the stubble. Occasionally they call to one another, a drawn-out melancholy bugle. The swans would have already disappeared from Suibara by the time Yoshio was a boy. Unlike his father, grandfather, and great-grandfather before him, Yoshio would have never heard the haunting wails of the whooper flock on Lake Hyoko when he walked out to the rice fields before dawn on a dark winter morning.

Years ago, when I began reading my father's letters, I wanted to imagine his war as fully as I could. After I learned the name inscribed on the mysterious flag, I wanted as well to imagine his foe. "It is not enough to just think about Yoshio, you must become Yoshio," the Swan Father might have said. Now, in this sheltered grove, I stand motionless and quiet, observing the rise and fall of my breath. Yoshio might have played here, I think to myself. I don't presume to become Yoshio, but eventually, he does come into focus.

In the December morning chill he wears only his thin navy-blue school uniform. His hair is cropped short and, without his school cap, his bare scalp is exposed and vulnerable. He shivers, stamps his feet.

Yoshio gazes through cedar boughs at rice paddies stretching miles toward the sharp dark contours of distant mountains. At the edge of the nearest field, unpicked fruits on a leafless persimmon shine like New Year's lanterns against the dull gray sky. From a gnarled branch, a vulture stares down on a flock of mallards.

The cedar grove is behind a small ancestor shrine on the Nakayama family farm, on the dirt road that leads out of Suibara. The weathered beams of the shrine are embellished with carved boars and dragons. The few chrysanthemums — pale pink, yellow, crimson — still bloom beside the modest torii gate weighted with winter snow.

Inside, on the altar, the family has left offerings for their ancestors — rice cakes wrapped in bamboo leaves, dried persimmons, a clay jar containing miso paste. Yoshio's stomach rumbles; he hasn't eaten since early morning, and even then the meal was sparse. Soon he'll cut across the fields and head home for a lunch of soba noodles and pickles, then go back to school. Or . . . maybe he won't. It could be one of those days he doesn't make it back to the classroom, lingering in his private world though he knows he'll be punished when he returns tomorrow morning.

Mrs. Nakayama, his elementary school teacher, used to plead with him to obey the rules. She was kind, like his own mother. "Don't you want to learn as much as possible, Yoshio-san?" she'd ask and then smile. "You must come every day if you want to go to university, if you want to be something else besides a farmer." Nakayama-sensei was understanding and easy. Onori-sensei, his current teacher, didn't hesitate to whack a student with his bamboo rod when necessary. Just yesterday, Yoshio's friend Tatue earned a beating because his lunch was wrapped in a newspaper that contained a photograph of the emperor. Juices from pickled daikon had dripped onto the emperor's left boot.

The emperor's photo was not something to be treated casually. Every morning at school they stood at attention to recite the Imperial Rescript, facing the special alcove where the emperor's portrait was displayed. In a special notebook at home, Yoshio kept photos of the emperor he'd clipped from newspapers. Among his favorites was one showing the emperor at Yasukuni Shrine, praying for fallen soldiers.

Someday soon, Yoshio will become a warrior for the emperor. He is confident of passing the conscription physical, that he will be a "Class A" soldier. He won't wait for the red envelope to be delivered to his house, like his brother Heijiro had. Yoshio makes a fist, flexes his arms. He is strong from years of farmwork, from chinning himself on the branches of the trees in the cedar grove.

This grove has long been one of his favorite places. He knows the spaces between the trees.

He knows the distance from the shrine to the closest edge of the rice field. How cedar cones feel in the palm of his hand — their shape and weight. He knows just how much effort it takes to lob one past the farthest tree; they make excellent ammunition. He's hidden here before to ambush his friends in their games of "Destroyer-Torpedo." He thinks through the rules: torpedoes beat battleships; destroyers beat torpedoes; light cruisers beat destroyers; heavy cruisers beat light cruisers.

Yoshio keeps his play rifle stashed behind some tombstones in a corner of the grove. A wet snow begins to fall, landing gently on his bare head, stinging his cheeks. He ignores it, digging out the rifle, its bamboo barrel fixed to the stock with sisal cord, and runs his hands over the smooth wood. He wishes it were real, like the ones he's seen soldiers carry while training at Takada Military Headquarters, just a few miles across the valley. Their crisp uniforms, the sound of their boots thudding on the road, impressed him at first sight. He remembers his very first glimpse of real soldiers — almost six years ago — on the drill field, when recruits trained for duty in Manchuria, after the China Incident.

He lays his rifle in its niche and begins to cover it carefully with cedar boughs, but before he finishes, he is distracted by a loud hum in the sky. Glancing up, he sees a glorious sight: a squadron of Youth Air Soldiers tipping their wings over

Suibara. A flyover! He can tell they are crossing over the schoolyard, showing off for the students returning from lunch. Yoshio forgets his hunger, his hesitation to return to the classroom, the noodles waiting for him at home, and sprints back toward the wooden school building in the center of town.

A few students stand in the yard, blue uniforms flecked with snow, staring up in wonder at the lucky flyers. Yoshio tilts his head toward the squadron above; he thinks he can see the pilots' faces. They look so proud.

Before the last plane has disappeared from the leaden sky, the school principal materializes on the front steps. He exhorts the lagging students to join the others already gathered in the assembly hall. Yoshio kicks off his shoes and rushes inside. No stove has been lit; the hall is freezing cold. The students sit in half-circle rows on the floor, facing the front of the room. The object of their focus: a radio placed on a simple wooden table, turned on full volume. The stirring cadence of "The Battleship March," the unofficial navy anthem, issues from its speaker. Crackling sounds. Then the stunning announcement: "News special. News special. Beginning this morning before dawn, the Imperial Japanese Army and Navy have opened hostilities with the United States and England in the Western Pacific." Yoshio hears the strange word "Honolulu." The principal, flushed and excited, exclaims, "Wonderful!" Onori-sensei shouts

269

out, "We really did it!" The students erupt into cheers.

Yoshio can hardly wait for the bell to ring, hardly wait to rendezvous with his friends at the Nakayama family shrine where they can now make plans for fighting a *real* war.

After he enlists, his friends and family will walk with him through the streets of Suibara to the train station. Before he departs for Takada military headquarters, they will all sign their names on his *yosegaki,* the white silk banner with the bright red circle, the one he will wear inside his helmet wherever he is sent, a talisman to protect against danger.

SELECTED BIBLIOGRAPHY

Bergerud, Eric. *Touched with Fire: The Land War in the South Pacific.* Penguin Books, New York, 1996.

Bix, Herbert P. *Hirohito and the Making of Modern Japan.* HarperCollins, New York, 2000.

Brainard, Cecilia Manguerra. *When the Rainbow Goddess Wept.* Dutton, New York, 1994.

Buruma, Ian. *The Wages of Guilt: Memories of War in Germany and Japan.* Penguin Books, New York, 1995.

Chang, Iris. *The Rape of Nanking: The Forgotten Holocaust of World War II.* BasicBooks, New York, 1997.

Cook, Haruko Taya, and Theodore F. Cook. *Japan at War: An Oral History.* New Press, New York, 1992.

Dower, John W. *War without Mercy: Race and Power in the Pacific War.* Pantheon Books, New York, 1986.

Dower, John W. *Japan in War and Peace: Selected Essays.* New Press, New York, 1993.

Dower, John W. *Embracing Defeat: Japan in the Wake of World War II.* W. W. Norton, New York, 1999.

Edgerton, Robert B. *Warriors of the Rising Sun: A History of the Japanese Military.* Westview Press, Boulder, Colorado, 1997.

Ehrenreich, Barbara. *Blood Rites: Origins and History of the Passions of War.* Henry Holt, New York, 1997.

Fahey, James J. *Pacific War Diary, 1942–1945: The Secret Diary of an American Sailor.* Houghton Mifflin, Boston, 1963.

Field, Norma. *In the Realm of a Dying Emperor: A Portrait of Japan at Century's End.* Pantheon Books, New York, 1991.

Fussell, Paul. *Thank God for the Atom Bomb and Other Essays.* Ballantine Books, New York, 1988.

Fussell, Paul. *Wartime: Understanding and Behavior in the Second World War.* Oxford University Press, New York, 1989.

Gibney, Frank (Ed.). *Sensō: The Japanese Remember the Pacific War (Letters to the Editor of* Asahi Shimbun*).* M. E. Sharpe, Armonk, New York, 1995.

Graves, Robert. *Good-bye to All That.* Anchor Doubleday, New York, 1985.

Gray, J. Glenn. *The Warriors: Reflections on Men in Battle.* University of Nebraska Press, Lincoln and London, 1970.

Griffin, Susan. *A Chorus of Stones: The Private Life of War.* Doubleday, New York, 1992.

Grossman, Lieutenant Colonel David. *On Killing: The Psychological Cost of Learning to Kill in War and Society*. Little Brown, New York, 1995.

Harris, David. *Our War: What We Did in Vietnam and What It Did to Us*. Random House, New York, 1996.

Hersey, John. *Hiroshima*. Alfred A. Knopf, New York, 1985.

Hillman, James. "Mars, Arms, Rams, Wars: On the Love of War," in *Nuclear Strategy and the Code of the Warrior: Faces of Mars and Shiva in the Crisis of Human Survival*. North Atlantic Books, Berkeley, 1984.

Hynes, Samuel. *The Soldiers' Tale: Bearing Witness to Modern War*. Viking Penguin, New York, 1997.

Karolevitz, Captain Robert F. (Ed.). *The 25th Division and World War 2*. Twenty-fifth Infantry Division, Baton Rouge, 1946.

Keegan, John. *A History of Warfare*. Random House, New York, 1993.

Keene, Donald. *On Familiar Terms: To Japan and Back, a Lifetime across Cultures*. Kodansha International, New York, 1996.

Lifton, Robert Jay, and Greg Mitchell. *Hiroshima in America: A Half Century of Denial*. Avon Books, New York, 1996.

Linderman, Gerald F. *The World within War: America's Combat Experience in World War II*. Free Press, New York, 1997.

Lomax, Eric. *The Railway Man: A POW's*

Searing Account of War, Brutality, and Forgiveness. W. W. Norton, New York, 1995.

Manchester, William. *Goodbye, Darkness: A Memoir of the Pacific War.* Little Brown, Boston, 1980.

Ōe, Kenzaburō. *Japan, the Ambiguous, and Myself: The Nobel Prize Speech and Other Lectures.* Kodansha International, Tokyo, 1995.

Ōe, Kenzaburō. *Hiroshima Notes*, trans. David L. Swain. Grove Press, New York, 1996.

Ōoka, Shōhei. *Fires on the Plain.* Charles E. Tuttle, Tokyo, 1957.

Ōoka, Shōhei. *Taken Captive: A Japanese POW's Story*, trans. Wayne P. Lammers. John Wiley & Sons, New York, 1996.

Rochlin, Fred. *Old Man in a Baseball Cap: A Memoir of World War II.* HarperCollins, New York, 1999.

Sano, Iwao Peter. *One Thousand Days in Siberia: The Odyssey of a Japanese-American POW.* University of Nebraska Press, Lincoln and London, 1997.

Shay, Jonathan. *Achilles in Vietnam: Combat Trauma and the Undoing of Character.* Atheneum, New York, 1994.

Shriver, Donald W. *An Ethic for Enemies: Forgiveness in Politics.* Oxford University Press, New York, 1995.

Sledge, E. B. *With the Old Breed: At Peleliu and Okinawa.* Oxford University Press, New York, 1990.

Smith, Robert Ross. *The United States Army in*

World War II, the War in the Pacific: Triumph in the Philippines. Office of the Chief of Military History, Department of the Army, Washington, D.C., 1963.

Treat, John Whittier. *Writing Ground Zero: Japanese Literature and the Atomic Bomb.* University of Chicago Press, Chicago, 1995.

Vance-Watkins, Lequita. *White Flash/Black Rain: Women of Japan Relive the Bomb.* Milkweed Editions, Minneapolis, 1995.

Young, Louise. *Japan's Total Empire: Manchuria and the Culture of Wartime Imperialism.* University of California Press, Berkeley, 1999.

ACKNOWLEDGMENTS

Many people have assisted me on this long journey.

Many thanks to Rika Ohara, for first translating the flag; John Mellana, who pointed me in the direction of John Dower's work; Howard Junker, who published my long poem about Yoshio's flag in his magazine *zyzzyva*; editors Susan Brenneman and Bret Israel at the *Los Angeles Times Magazine*, who gave me the assignment to Japan; Paul Freireich at the *New York Times* travel section for his invaluable sleuthing; and Donna Frazier, who edited my article for the *Los Angeles Times Magazine* and in the process became a friend and invaluable guide.

Thanks to my wonderful family — to Florence Hamrol, a memorist herself; to Matthew Solomon, who provided many details from his memory; to Jennifer Solomon, who made the scrapbook of newspaper clippings about her grandfather's stint in the Pacific; to Larry Steinman, who asked critical questions and read the poem at Passover; to Ruth Solomon, for her encouragement and insights; and to Ken Steinman for stories and support.

For straight talk, nudging, notes on the manuscript, and practical advice about Japan, many thanks to Alan Brown. Thanks to Amy Morita for being the liaison with the Japanese Ministry of Health and Welfare. Lindy Hough and Judith Nies both offered detailed read-throughs of the manuscript and gave helpful suggestions. Thanks to Adam Hochschild for inspiration and encouragement, and to Professor John Dower for the afternoon he spent with me, for taking my project seriously.

Thanks to Susan Banyas, Charlotte Hildebrand, Irene Borger, Erica Clark, for listening and sharing their stories. Thanks to the following for various support over the years of writing: Steve Clorfeine, Anne Dubuisson, Suzanne Edison, Ginnah Howard, Sally Kaplan, Joan Kreiss, Sarah Jacobus, Meredith Monk, Anna Valentina Murch, Regina O'Melveney, Dennis Palumbo, Roger Perlmutter, Wendy Perron, Rob and Barbara Pressman, Chris Rauschenbert, Olga Serova, Jim Siegel, Don Singer, Janet Stein, Laura Stickney, Beth Thielen, and Ellen Zweig.

Other helpers provided translation and information. Yukiko Amaya, Nancy Beckman, Gen Watanabe, Chiyoko Osborne, and Salud Ilao — many thanks.

Special thanks to Centrum Foundation in Port Townsend, Washington, for providing the environment in which my father's letters first came alive; to the California Community Foundation for the Brody Literary Fellowship, which facilitated my first trip to Japan; and to Blue Mountain Center for the blessing of a month of peaceful writing and thinking. The good folks at the Japanese National Tourist Organization helped me find my way around Japan, and provided assistance with lodging and rail travel. Thanks also to International House in Tokyo, for their formidable library. The Library Foundation of Los Angeles accommodated my travel and writing retreats and offered a supportive atmosphere in which to work. My colleague Toby Dell held the fort in my absence. The librarians and staff at the Los Angeles Public Library daily manage to work miracles, and I thank them for their assistance.

In Japan, the Shimizu family and their neighbors and friends received me with love in their hearts. Many thanks to Mayor Ikarashi and Mihara Kenzo for their many kindnesses. I am indebted to Mrs. Seito, Mrs. Nakamura, Mr. Watanabe, and Mr. Abe for sharing their stories. In Hiroshima, thanks to the Kurokami family for their delightful hospitality, especially to Shoji Kurokami for being my guide. Thanks to Marcy and Lauren Homer and Chitaru Satake at the Ministry of Health and Welfare.

Thanks to my "muses," all World War II vets and all very wise men: Sylvan Katz, Peter Lomenzo, Baldwin Eckel, and Fred Rochlin. They shared their difficult experiences with me,

278

and accepted my naivete with grace and generosity. Their stories have moved me deeply and I am honored to help share them with others.

There are four more people without whom this whole project would not have been possible: Betsy Amster, my wonderful agent who is also a fine editor, has been patient, prodding, enthusiastic, and honest during these many years. She always believed that "Yoshio" would be a book and encouraged me to take whatever time was necessary to finish it. Antonia Fusco, my editor at Algonquin Books, recognized this story in the rough and made it a far better telling. Working with her is a privilege and a pleasure. Masako Hayakawa was more than a translator. She was my cultural guide, a true friend and stalwart ally who made real sacrifices to assist me. I am deeply indebted to her as well as to her husband, Professor Norio Hayakawa, for sharing his story. Finally, my deepest gratitude to my husband, Lloyd Hamrol, who accompanied me to the mountaintop, took photographs while suffering the flu, cooked dinners, edited, brainstormed, suffered my doubts, weathered my manias, fed the cat, listened to dreams, offered structural insights and unconditional love.

The employees of Thorndike Press hope you have enjoyed this Large Print book. All our Large Print titles are designed for easy reading, and all our books are made to last. Other Thorndike Press Large Print books are available at your library, through selected bookstores, or directly from the publishers.

For more information about titles, please call:

(800) 223-1244
(800) 223-6121

To share your comments, please write:

Publisher
Thorndike Press
295 Kennedy Memorial Drive
Waterville, ME 04901